Y0-BQT-048

The *Sexy Little Book* of

SEX
GAMES

Ava Cadell, Ph.D., Ed.D.

ALPHA

A member of Penguin Group (USA) Inc.

ALPHA BOOKS

Published by the Penguin Group

Penguin Group (USA) Inc., 375 Hudson Street, New York, New York 10014, USA

Penguin Group (Canada), 90 Eglinton Avenue East, Suite 700, Toronto, Ontario M4P 2Y3, Canada
(a division of Pearson Penguin Canada Inc.)

Penguin Books Ltd., 80 Strand, London WC2R 0RL, England

Penguin Ireland, 25 St. Stephen's Green, Dublin 2, Ireland (a division of Penguin Books Ltd.)

Penguin Group (Australia), 250 Camberwell Road, Camberwell, Victoria 3124, Australia (a division of
Pearson Australia Group Pty. Ltd.)

Penguin Books India Pvt. Ltd., 11 Community Centre, Panchsheel Park, New Delhi—110 017, India

Penguin Group (NZ), 67 Apollo Drive, Rosedale, North Shore, Auckland 1311, New Zealand (a division of
Pearson New Zealand Ltd.)

Penguin Books (South Africa) (Pty.) Ltd., 24 Sturdee Avenue, Rosebank, Johannesburg 2196, South Africa

Penguin Books Ltd., Registered Offices: 80 Strand, London WC2R 0RL, England

Copyright © 2012 by Ava Cadell, Ph.D., Ed.D.

International Standard Book Number: 978-1-61564-142-0
Library of Congress Catalog Card Number: 2011910190

14 13 12   8 7 6 5 4 3 2

Interpretation of the printing code: The rightmost number of the first series of numbers is the year of
the book's printing; the rightmost number of the second series of numbers is the number of the book's
printing. For example, a printing code of 12-1 shows that the first printing occurred in 2012.

Printed in the United States of America

Note: This publication contains the opinions and ideas of its author. It is intended to provide helpful and
informative material on the subject matter covered. It is sold with the understanding that the author and
publisher are not engaged in rendering professional services in the book. If the reader requires personal
assistance or advice, a competent professional should be consulted.

The author and publisher specifically disclaim any responsibility for any liability, loss, or risk, personal or
otherwise, which is incurred as a consequence, directly or indirectly, of the use and application of any of
the contents of this book.

Trademarks: All terms mentioned in this book that are known to be or are suspected of being trademarks
or service marks have been appropriately capitalized. Alpha Books and Penguin Group (USA) Inc. cannot
attest to the accuracy of this information. Use of a term in this book should not be regarded as affecting the
validity of any trademark or service mark.

Most Alpha books are available at special quantity discounts for bulk purchases for sales promotions,
premiums, fund-raising, or educational use. Special books, or book excerpts, can also be created to fit
specific needs.

For details, write: Special Markets, Alpha Books, 375 Hudson Street, New York, NY 10014.

This book is dedicated to my husband Peter Knecht who's kept a playful, mischievous quality for the past 20 years that makes him fun to play sex games with.

Contents

Introduction

This book is not for couples that take sex too seriously. It's for any adult—gay, bi, or straight—who wants to make sex more playful, passionate, and unpredictable. Whether you're single, dating, cohabitating, or wed, you'll find a plethora of sex games that will make you laugh, talk, touch, tease, and truly connect with your partner. You'll find games you can play to create more romance, seduction, arousal, sensuality, intimacy, and kink, but be warned as there are countless games that are so sexually graphic, they may result in multiple orgasms for guys and gals. Ultimately, this book can transform your love life by giving you the skills to be a great lover who is memorably exciting and fun. Couples who play together, stay together!

Extras

Enjoy extra tips and tricks throughout the book in these sidebars that will make your sex games even more fun:

Definitions of words to help you expand your sexy vocabulary;

Suggestions to enhance your sex games with more props, people, and other playful ideas;

Fun facts that can make you the life of any party;

And cautionary tips on what not to do to make your sex games safe and pleasurable.

Acknowledgments

Dr. Hernando Chaves, the kinkiest Sexologist I know; Brian Pellham, CEO of Kheper Games; Lei Lei Sun, Director of Product Development for Hustler Toys; Tamara Bell, CEO of Home Pleasure Party Plan Assoc.; Shelly Barnum, my assistant; and Loveology University Honor students: Tiffany Juterbock, Susan Compton, Kim Varner, and Angel Lowe.

1

Fun with Foreplay

Foreplay is the perfect playground for lovers to get each other relaxed and ready for great sex. Foreplay is fun playtime without intercourse, so you could describe it as flirtations, sensual play, frisky play, or even "outercourse."

In this chapter, we'll explore a variety of foreplay games you can play to tease and tantalize your lover. Have fun with them and discuss with your lover which ones are worthy of a repeat performance. You'll find that foreplay can be your prelude to great sex or even become an unforgettable main event.

Flirtations

Flirtation games are a perfect setup for a night of memorable sex with your lover. They create romance, instill sexual confidence, and maintain sexual chemistry between the two of you. Flirting in a variety of different ways creates a connection of desire and mystery leading the way to pleasurable heights.

Mirror, Mirror on the Wall

This game can become a fun ritual that will keep your love life lusty. Take your favorite colored lipstick, a bar of soap, or shaving cream to write something sexy on the bathroom mirror for your lover to see. Or simply tape a note to the mirror that says something erotic, such as, "I want you now." Have fun surprising each other by leaving notes with different messages every day in different places—in her purse or his wallet, in the car, or in a pocket.

Memory Maker

Create a romantic scrapbook with your lover by collecting some of your couple memorabilia—love letters, cards, event tickets, menus, and matchbooks from places you've been together—and enjoy walking down memory lane and reminiscing as you paste them into a book. Then test each other to see who can remember the correct dates to write under each item. Remember to have fun with it and not make it overly serious, and let the sparks of your fond memories lead to the making of more memorable moments.

One-Night Stand

Have a one-night stand with your partner by going to a public place and pretending you've never met. Flirt and seduce each other with the intention of having the kind of naughty, uninhibited passionate sex with a one-night stand you know you'll never see again. If you're at a bar that has a dance floor, party and make out like two high school kids. The game is to see if you can pull it off without anyone suspecting that you know each other.

To make your one-night stand even more exciting, ladies, wear a Hustler Toy wireless Bang Bang Bullet in your underwear and give your lover the controller.

Romance Journal

Pretend to be a best-selling romance novelist and write down lots of romantic activities in a journal. It could be anything from throwing rose petals on the bed, a candlelit bubble bath, or collecting pebbles while taking a romantic walk on a beach, to riding a motorcycle together through the countryside, skinny dipping in a private lagoon, or watching a sexy movie together—whatever your definition of romance is. Let your partner read your journal and act as your editor to add and edit his or her ideas to your romantic activities. Be sure to act some, or all, of them out.

Trinket Surprises

Surprise each other by giving little gifts for no special reason. A single flower, some candy, lip balm, a new CD, or even this book will let your lover know that you are thinking about them in a sexy way. The game is to see who can surprise their partner at the most unexpected times with the most unusual little gifts. It's not the price tag of the gifts that count, it's the thought of giving a little something unexpected to show you're thinking of each other.

Pubic Styles

Shaving your lover's pubic hair can be fun and very sexy foreplay. Take turns shaving each other to see who can create the most imaginative design. Some popular shapes are a triangle, a landing strip, and a heart. Also, the trust you and your lover share to shave each other makes it a highly erotic experience.

All Day Flirtations

Call and text your lover during the day with compliments like, "You're so hot, I love the way you touch me," and with ideas on how you want to make love tonight like, "Let's do it with the lights on, I want you to undress me," and so on.

Sensual Foreplay

Sensual play is all about playing with the five senses in different ways and drawing attention to your lover's sensuousness. These games all have seductive pleasures to please you and your lover.

Sensational Sense

Find five items that enhance and heighten each one of your senses, so ten items total. For the sense of sight, you can get fresh cut flowers or lingerie. For the sense of smell, try scented candles or incense. For sound, play romantic music or get some wind chimes. The sense of taste can be enhanced with chocolates or fresh fruit. And the sense of touch can be heightened by the use of feathers or massage oil. If you both choose the same thing for one of the senses, the first one to exchange it with something else gets to have a sensual massage first.

Limo Love

Rent a limo for the night and bring along a bottle of a bubbly, fresh strawberries dipped in chocolate, and set the mood with sexy music. If you tell the limo driver that you're celebrating a special event, he or she will leave you two alone. Now that you've got your privacy you can truly enjoy the ride making out in that big, back seat like a couple of celebrities. But don't stop there, get your money's worth by teasing, tantalizing, and undressing each other. The winner of this game is the most daring lover in the back of that limo, and the loser has to tip the driver.

Passion Wheel

Draw a circle and then divide it up into 8 to 12 parts. Then each of you writes on the parts what activities you want to do to enhance your relationship equally. For example: cuddling, kissing, caressing, oral sex, role-playing, massage, phone sex, etc. Then take turns choosing one activity to do from the Passion Wheel each day. You can also play this game by pointing to an activity while blindfolded.

Disrobing Desire

See how long it takes each of you to slowly disrobe each other and appreciate every new area of skin that gets exposed, teasing as you go to create incredible sexual anticipation. Kiss, caress, and nibble sexual and nonsexual areas as you give compliments to your lover. Whoever takes the longest is the winner.

Making love while still dressed builds more arousal, so caress and lick her through her bra or panties and fondle and lick him while unzipping his pants, but don't take them off.

Kidnapper

With your lover's permission, blindfold him or her and drive them to a secret sexy destination, giving little clues about where you're going along the way. If they guess where you are going, then they can take the blindfold off, but if they can't, they must leave it on until you take it off.

Strip Poker Dinner

The best way to play strip poker is to surprise your lover by playing the game while dinner is in the oven. Once the game is underway, be prepared to lose one article of clothing with each hand that you lose. Everybody wins when you're both naked and the mood changes from competitive to sexy. Make sure you serve and eat dinner in the nude to top off the evening.

Frisky Foreplay

Foreplay doesn't always have to be gentle or slow to trigger romance or sex. Foreplay can be lively and silly so you and your lover can laugh and have fun playing together.

Tickle War

Tickle each other's armpits, bare feet, ribs, and tummy until one of you cannot take anymore and surrenders. You can use your fingers, a feather, or a brush on your lover's tickle spots.

Pillow Fight

Have a pillow fight on the bed and try to knock each other down. Whoever scores three knockdowns is the winner, and the loser must masturbate for the winner.

Naked Wrestling

Challenge your lover to a naked wrestling match, going over the rules before you begin. Wrestle each other gently, not rough and no biting or hair pulling, for three rounds of two minutes each. The first one to straddle and pin their lover's arms down is the winner and the prize is that he or she gets to have an orgasm first.

Before you start tickling, wrestling, or pillow fighting with your lover, agree upon a safe word that means "Stop Now!" You can use "Red" for the traffic light or anything else that will be taken seriously.

Animal Magnetism

Get into an animal posture and attitude by making the sounds and movements of your chosen animal. You can be a snake and slither all over your lover, a monkey playfully exploring your lover, a cat who snuggles, or any other animal you choose. If your lover guesses the animal that you are, then he or she gets to choose what kind of animal he wants you to be in bed.

Stripper Tease

Visuals play a big role in foreplay, especially for guys, so a woman who wears sexy clothes, high heels, and naughty lingerie is a big turn on, but taking it off seductively is the hottest kind of foreplay for a man. Women enjoy seeing a man taking his clothes off, too, so take turns doing a strip tease for each other. To make this game even more fun, tip your lover generously by sliding lots of bills in their pants, shorts, bra, panties, or G-string. And remember, a lap dance is extra!

Saving Water

Surprise your lover in the shower when they least expect it and join them for a hot, steamy shower together. Take turns giving each other a rub down with soap or a sexy smelling body wash. The thicker the lather the better, so you can press your slippery, wet bodies up against each other and slide them together like a human washcloth.

Outercourse Games

Outercourse is exciting foreplay without having intercourse that can even result in orgasms. With limitless pleasure possibilities, these games are meant to promote passion without going all the way.

Mutual Masturbation

Leave your inhibitions behind and face each other as you touch yourselves at the same time. Be sure to look at your lover while you're playing with yourself because this game is a staring contest while you masturbate, and the loser is the one who looks away first. The winner gets to choose their favorite sexy movie to watch together.

Show and Tell

Demonstrate on any part of your body and tell your lover, "I want to show you where and how I like to be touched." Then show him or her and express exactly how it is most enjoyable for you. To be sure that your lover has been paying attention, ask them to show you what they have learned. You can grade them on their skill and if they get high marks, then reward them by asking them to Show and Tell you about their body.

The Watcher

After a romantic dinner, gradually move your party of two into the bedroom. With the lights down low and soft music playing in the background, flip a coin to determine who is going to be the watcher, then he or she takes a seat on a chair while the other person reclines on the bed. The watcher then tells his or her lover what to do while they watch. There are no rules, so go for it and tell him or her to talk dirty, strip, climax, or do anything you desire.

The Weekender

Clear your schedule because the only work you're going to be
doing over this weekend is pleasing your lover in between the
sheets. It's okay to keep the TV and DVD in the bedroom, but
only if you are going to throw in an adult movie to liven things
up. Flip a coin to determine who will be making or ordering
food to eat in bed. You can have it delivered to your door, just
don't forget to put on some clothes first.

> The rules for spending the weekend in bed include
> turning your phone off and not talking about any
> problems or everyday concerns. If someone breaks
> the rules, then he or she gets a spanking.

Sack Jack

Just as you would play Black Jack, assign one partner the dealer
role while the other is the player. Rather than betting money,
bet on foreplay favors such as kisses, caresses, and licks. You can
add to the fun by including other rules such as if either partner
makes 21, then the other partner has to remove an article of
clothing, or if either partner "busts" (goes over 21) they have to
initiate another foreplay game.

Jenga Gone Wild

Buy a Jenga game that is made of a light colored wood and
use a Sharpie to write in foreplay requests. You can write one
sentence per block such as, slow dance with me. Set up the game
with your newly decorated blocks in a random order with some

sentences facing in, out, sideways; sometimes it's fun to see or not see what you are about to choose. If someone successfully takes out the block, then the other person has to complete the assigned task in no more than 30 seconds. If a partner causes all of the blocks to fall down, then the other partner can choose any random three blocks and have their partner fulfill their foreplay fantasy.

Penis Play

Ask your lover where he would put his penis if he were engaging in femoral, gluteal, popliteal, or spinal sex rubbing. For each one that he gets right, he can actually do the deed. Here are the answers:

- Femoral Sex: rubbing between the thighs

- Gluteal Sex: rubbing between the butt cheeks

- Popliteal Sex: rubbing behind the semi-bent knee

- Spinal Sex: rubbing between the neck and shoulder

Petal Play

You will need to have a fresh flower with petals like an orchid, rose, or sunflower in advance of this game. Begin playing once your lover is lying on a bed naked with a blindfold covering his or her eyes. Then tease them by gently caressing their body with the petals of the flower and ask if they can guess what kind of flower it is. Do your best to bring them to a full body orgasm before guessing the flower.

You can reenact the sexy scene from the movie *40 Days and 40 Nights* where Josh Hartnett caresses Shannyn Sossamon's body sensuously with flower petals until she reaches an orgasm.

20 Minutes of Outercourse

The rules of this game are that you can do anything sexual with your partner except have intercourse for 20 minutes without stopping. To be sure that you get your full 20 minutes, set an alarm clock.

4 Play

Enjoy these four titillating games to get your juices flowing: Foreplay Dice, where you roll dice to perform sensual actions on your lover; Foreplay Fortune is a game where you and your lover use cards to act out fun fantasies; The Wheel of Pleasure has a spinner to play and perform sexy activities; and in S,E,X Marks the Spot game, you spin the sex top and try to make it stop on the body part of your lover you want to satisfy. 4 Play is made by Kheper Games and is available online and at all Hustler stores.

Group Foreplay Games

If you have some close open-minded friends who want to have some adult fun, then these games will rev them up and send them home ready for action.

Hunters and Prey

Nominate one person to be the prey and have them sit in the middle of a circle blindfolded. The rest of the group are the hunters who must touch the prey sensually. The prey's goal is to identify who each hunter is that has touched him or her. If a hunter is successfully identified, he or she becomes the new prey.

Group Strip Poker

Begin playing strip poker to remove clothing, then up the stakes by adding foreplay activities like kissing, dirty talk, sucking, massaging, dry humping, and spanking.

Sexy Truth or Dare

Lose your inhibitions and get ready to reveal your dirtiest secrets as you ask the most intimate questions like, "Who would you like to cum inside," and dares like, "I dare you to sit on so and so's face naked."

Foreplay Dice

You can play this game with two regular dice, some paper, and a pen. Before you begin, write down a list of six erogenous zones that everyone agrees they want stimulated such as the neck, nipples, thighs, butt, pussy, and balls. Then write a second list of actions that you all want performed on your body such as kissing, licking, pinching, blowing, slapping, and sucking. Take turns rolling the dice and coordinating the body part with one dice and the action with the other dice.

Closet Foreplay

Draw straws or names from a hat for this game to determine which two people go into a dark closet for three minutes of foreplay. Use a timer so that everyone can see when the time is up.

2

Food Games and Aphrodisiacs

Food and sex are two of the greatest pleasures known to mankind, and both appetites need to be fulfilled. So get ready to feast on love foods and aphrodisiacs that can boost your sex drive and spice up your sex life.

In this chapter, you'll discover countless love food games that can be incorporated into foreplay, seduction, and sexual performance to intensify your orgasms.

Foods for the Mood

These foreplay foods send blood to the sex organs to get you and your lover in the mood. The seduction foods heighten your arousal level even more and performance enhancer foods increase the intensity of orgasms.

Foreplay Foods

Chili Pepper Madness

Hot chili peppers get the face flushing, heart pumping, pores sweating, and blood flowing toward the genitals. Have a contest to see who can eat the most chili peppers. The winner gets to have their orgasm first.

Chocolate Delight

Chocolate includes a plant substance called phytosterol that mimics human sex hormones. Share a box of assorted chocolates with your lover by selecting and feeding them to each other. If you guess the right kind of chocolate, you get a kiss but if you're wrong, you get bitten.

Apple Bobbing

Apples are known as the fruit of temptation since the beginning of time, and they are filled with vitamins, minerals, and enzymes that stimulate sexual desire. See who can catch an apple floating in water with their teeth the quickest. The winner gets a lap dance.

Apple Bobbing can be a fun and sexy game to do with a close group of friends over a big bowl of fruit punch.

Naked Sushi

Ginger increases blood flow to the genitals in both men and women. Fresh ginger compliments sushi, so this is a perfect opportunity to eat sushi off your lover's naked body, and don't forget to add the ginger on top.

Seduction Foods

Oyster Inhale

Oysters contain zinc, an essential mineral for men needed for sperm production and it releases testosterone in men and women. Take turns sucking an oyster from its shell. The person who does it the most seductively wins the sex position of their choice.

Shrimp Feeder

Shrimp is high in iodine, which is needed by the thyroid gland that regulates energy, including sexual energy. Each partner should take a turn feeding the other shrimp. Be sure to lick, suck, and nibble the shrimp as well as your lover's fingers. The one who is the most sexual wins one free fantasy.

Olive Lipstick

Green olives are believed to make men more virile while black ones can increase sex drive for women. Slowly outline your lips with an olive then give your partner an olive lipstick kiss. You can also have your partner remove the pimento filling from a green olive and put it on his or her finger, then use it to outline your lips before sharing a kiss.

Tomato Pasty Sensation

Tomatoes are known as "love apples," and in early times were forbidden by Puritans because of its reputation as a potent sexual stimulant. Slice a tomato and attach it to your nipples like a pasty and have your partner slowly eat it off, sucking and nibbling your nipple along the way.

Performance Foods

Peter Pumpkin Eater

Pumpkin pie is the top contender to increase penile blood flow by an average of 40 percent faster. Spread a slice of pumpkin pie between your lover's thighs and slowly eat it all up before you enter your next intercourse.

Spend 15 to 20 minutes licking up the pumpkin pie between the thighs and wait until your partner can't stand it any longer before you move on to what you want to do next.

Bind with Vines

Licorice contains plant estrogens and stimulates the sex glands, bringing oxygen to the female genitals 40 percent faster. Tie licorice ropes around your partner's penis as you perform oral sex on him. For your reward, you get to have your orgasm first.

Cinnamon Delight

Cinnamon has a sweet, spicy flavor, and its aroma has been used to aid in the treatment of impotence and is proven to be sexually stimulating for men. Dust a few drops of cinnamon behind your ear, on your nipple, and around genitals so that your lover can have a tasty treat when they explore your body with their tongue.

Herb Erotica

Basil is considered the sacred herb of India; it awakens the senses, stimulates blood flow, and relieves fatigue. Rub basil over both you and your lover's bodies and cuddle together inhaling the fresh scent. The first one to get aroused gets to start the lovemaking session with any sexual activity of their choice.

Stalk of Passion

Celery contains androsterone, a powerful male hormone released through sweat glands to attract women. Place a celery stalk in your mouth and try to prevent your lover from eating the other end by moving it around with your teeth and lips so that he or she has a hard time reaching it. If he or she can catch the celery stalk, they win an erotic massage.

Shapely Food Games

Many roots, vegetables, and fruits became known as aphrodisiacs simply because their shapes were designed by nature as a clue to their use. Find as many foods as you can that resemble the sexual organs and then use them to tease your lover. Here are a few examples.

Banana

Lick, suck, deep-throat, and nibble on a banana to give your man an erotic visual sensation of what you can do with his penis.

Carrot

Put a condom on this phallus of the vegetable kingdom and pleasure yourself with it in front of your lover.

Clam

Lick around the edges of the clam as if it was a vulva and then slowly suck on it before slurping it down your throat. Then do the same to her.

Fig

Spread the fig apart with your fingers as if spreading the labia and use your mouth to make out with it as you suck and nibble the fresh fruit sensually. Then you can have the real thing.

Other female-shaped foods include pears, mussels, mangos, peaches, nectarines, pomegranates, passion fruits, and artichokes.

Male-shaped, or phallic, foods include asparagus, cucumbers, squash, zucchinis, parsnips, turnips, licorices, celery, and leeks.

Body Food Games

These food games have added nourishment, exercise, and fun all rolled into one. You'll not only enjoy the food, but you'll enjoy how you get to eat it.

Sploshing

Fulfill your wildest fantasies by covering your lover's body with messy food such as mashed potatoes, gravy, spaghetti and meatballs, ice cream, custard, baked beans, and peanut butter. Then eat it off. At worst you'll need to practice sponge bath techniques. At best, you'll never need to wash any dishes.

The word *Sploshing* is defined as a Wet and Messy Fetishism, whereby applying messy foods and substances onto another person is sexually arousing.

Body Art

Turn your lover's body into a canvas by eating your favorite foods off of your lover's body. The game is to paint a scene on any part of your lover's body with the food, and if they guess what it is you can eat it off. If they can't guess what it is, then you must continue to paint until they can describe your artistic masterpiece.

Fun foods for body painting include chocolate sauce, whipped cream, peanut butter, jam, syrup, honey, and all kinds of berries.

Hide the Honey

Decide who is going to be the hider and who is going to be the seeker. The hider will be the receiver of pleasure lying naked on the bed while the seeker will put on a blindfold. The hider must hide a dab of honey somewhere on their body and tell their lover to find it without using their hands.

Ice Landing

Begin with ice and rub it up and down your lover's spine, behind their ears and down the neck, around the breasts, on the inside of the thighs, and so on. See if they can handle this until the ice melts.

Kool Whip

See who can write the word "sex" with a can of whipping cream on their lover's body the fastest. The winner gets to lick it off.

Slip and Slide

Pour flavored gelatin into the showerhead, turn on the hot shower, and take the most delightful gooey, slippery, and sensual shower of your life.

Artichoke Arousal

Make one artichoke for both of you to share. Every time you pick off an artichoke leaf, before you nibble on it, give your lover a sexy treat. Remove a piece of your clothing, give them a sensual kiss, or say something sexy—use your imagination to come up with little treats. Now it's your lover's turn. By the time you reach the heart, you'll both be feeling very good about each other and may be too aroused for the main course.

The Ice Creamer

Take turns as one of you stands above the other person, who lies down with an ice-cream cone in their mouth. The person standing must drop ice-cream toppings like nuts, chocolate drops, sprinkles, and gummy candy on top of the cone. The person with the best-looking cone topping is the winner and they get to eat the ice cream off their lover's body.

Liquor Licker

Pour your favorite liquor or liqueur over your lover's body (not in it) and lick it off planting extra passionate kisses, licks, and sucks. Then kiss and see if your lover can guess your liquor or liqueur of choice.

Be careful to keep foods and liquids out of the vagina since they can cause infections.

Sex Food Party

This game is fun for a group of friends who love to eat and play. Tell everyone to bring a food that most resembles their sexual personality. For example, one person might bring some chili or hot salsa to symbolize a spicy sexy personality. Display all of the food on a table and give each guest a piece of paper with a list of everybody's name. The object of the game is to guess who goes with which food. Everyone will write the food next to the person's name it most resembles. Then, one by one each person reveals their food and describes how it resembles their sexual

personality. Whoever has the most correct answers is the winner.
The prize can be a box of chocolates and a sex toy.

Romantic Food Games

Food and romance go together quite nicely, and can lead to
memorable sexual encounters. Use these food games to arouse
and seduce your lover in a whole new way.

Eating In

Surprise your lover with a romantic meal at home and seduce
him or her by serving them naked, feeding each other, and
savoring each bite. Whether you prepare breakfast, lunch, dinner, or just a snack, use a variety of flavors and textures beauti-
fully presented so that you have lots to play with.

Morning Love Potion

Rather than starting your morning with a cup of coffee, put
your body in lovemaking mode with a smoothie of fresh berries,
orange, bananas, and honey. To make it even more exciting,
serve the smoothie to your lover in a fancy wine glass and come
dressed or undressed for the occasion. Use the smoothie for
foreplay and see who gets aroused first.

Breast Fruits

Grapefruits, oranges, and other citrus fruits resemble a woman's
breasts. Take the fruit of your choice and lick and suck it sensuously as if it was a beautiful woman's breasts. Whoever gets
aroused first will also get to be eaten first.

Sexy Picnic

Take a lovely picnic basket filled with your favorite finger foods, such as fresh fruits, vegetables, and an assortment of sweets, to a park, beach, or forest. Put a blindfold on your partner and have them guess what foods you feed them. If you're feeling adventurous in the great outdoors, make your partner taste them on different parts of your body.

Designer Dinner

The purpose of this Designer Dinner is to achieve total decadence, uninhibited indulgence of your favorite foods combined with wild and wonderful sex games, and to create an erotic keepsake menu for your lover. Make some of the items to share with your lover, and remove a piece of clothing after each course. Here's a sample menu:

Foreplay

Phallic Endives Salad with Passion Dressing

Cheeky Chicken Salad with Tantalizing Toasted Almonds

Erotic Tuna Tartar on Lusty Lotus Chips

Saucy Split Pea Soup with Fresh Cream

Seduction

Erogenous Chicken Brochette and Virgin Vegetables

Sexy Beef with Sizzling Hot Chili Peppers

Afterglow Mandarin Glazed Duck Tossed with Sensuous Noodles

Seductive Seared Salmon with Amorous Arugula Salad

Climax

Aphrodite's Apple Pie

Fetish Chocolate Mousse

Sadistic Mini Key Limes

Multi-Climactic Cookies

My Love Food Sign

You and your partner should select one love food each that signals to your partner that you want to have sex. For example, she may select a chocolate and he may select a banana. When either partner wants to signal their desire to have sex, just place your signal item on the bed pillow.

Shop and Top

Take a trip to the local grocery store and purchase sauces and syrups you and your lover will enjoy trickling onto nipples, thighs, back, neck, toes, fingers, and other body parts. Using index cards, write the name of the toppings purchased, one on each card. Shuffle the cards and have your lover pick a card. The card picked is the flavor for the night.

Lust on the Rocks

Take turns putting a piece of ice into your mouth between your teeth or lips to see how long you can keep it in as you run it all across your partner's body. The person who keeps the ice in play the longest, until it completely melts or as close to that point as possible, wins the game.

Letter of the Lay

Write each letter of the alphabet on index cards then shuffle them up. Take turns picking one card a day and whatever letter you pick determines what kind of food you must bring into your next lovemaking session. Example: Apple, Butter, Cream, Dates, Endive, Flour, and so on. What you do with the food is up to your sexual desire of the day.

Baste Your Lover

Heat up some gravy so that it's nice and warm (but not too hot!), and then put it in a turkey baster. Use your gravy-filled baster to draw a picture or just drizzle it on your lover's body, then slowly lick it all off.

Naked Chef

Cook together in the nude and use kitchen utensils to arouse your lover—use a spatula for a light spank or a pastry brush to add oil for an erotic massage. (Be careful when using the stove or oven to not burn any delicate body parts!)

Herbs of Passion

Jasmine, rosemary, and sage are said to increase arousal when rubbed on the skin. Applying them to erogenous zones, such as the neck and to stress-carrying areas such as the back, lower tension and can stir sensuous feelings. Use the various herbs to see how you and your lover's senses are aroused and discover which one sparks your passion.

Tasty Wear

Surprise your lover with some candy cuffs that you can nibble off their wrists. How about some edible undies, stretchy candy cock-rings, nipple tassels, or even a sweet candy whip? All of these edibles plus erotic chocolate pussies, breasts, butts, and penises are available for a fun date where you can eat your way to sexual heaven. Visit www.chocolatefantasies.com to find these edible delights.

3

Sex Talk Games

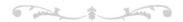

In this chapter, you'll learn how to make erotic talk a natural part of your love life through imaginative games to play face-to-face, and by phone, video, audio, and text that will leave your partner breathless.

By using sounds, words, and phrases that excite your partner, you can bring greater passion to your lovemaking and even open up doors of communication, which may have previously been closed.

Sounds of Sex

Making sounds of pleasure during sex is a quick and easy way to let your partner know that you're having a great time.

Aural Sex

Record your next lovemaking session and play it back to hear the noises you both make, and who makes the most. Common sounds of sex are moaning, groaning, panting, giggling, growling, screaming, gasping, laughing, whimpering, sighing, howling, and heavy breathing. The winner of making the most sounds gets to choose his or her favorite position.

When you release sounds during sex, you release increased sexual energy and you can experience more intense orgasms.

Sex Tones

Depending on your voice tone, volume, tempo, and high or low pitch, you can turn someone on (or off). Take turns saying "I want you now" using theses various vocal tones:

- Gentle
- Deep
- Husky
- Slow

- Whispery
- Excited
- Aggressive
- Baby talk

Then tell your partner which vocal tones turn you on the most.

Role Play

Throw away your inhibitions and role play different personalities to keep your partner guessing who he or she is going to have sex with next. Talk about which personalities you each like the most.

The Porn Star

Make loud exaggerated noises in response to what your lover is doing and praise him or her with "It's so big," or "You're so hot." Throw in explicit four letter words as you pick up speed and keep repeating, "Yes, yes, yes, harder, more" as you shake your head and thrash your body like a porn star.

The Director

You are in control, so give orders to your lover as he or she goes down on you and say, "Now you're hitting the right spot, that's how I need it." If they stop, say "I didn't say stop." Keep directing your lover in different ways.

The Romantic

Whisper in your lover's ear, "It feels so good when you're inside me or when I'm inside you. I love you." Sensually shout your partner's name during orgasm.

The Novice

Act like a sexual beginner wanting to please your lover. Ask for guidance and validation with phrases like, "Tell me how you like to be sucked or licked, I want to give you the best possible orgasm," and "How am I doing?"

The Slave

Be a willing lover who wants to be controlled by a Master or Mistress, by saying, "I've been very bad and need to be punished."

If you're a businessman or woman during the day, don't let that stop you from being a Porn Star in bed. It's also not unusual for professional authoritarians to enjoy relinquishing their power between the sheets to become the Slave or a Novice.

Sensual Chatter

By using certain words to heighten your lover's senses you can arouse his or her desire and deepen the intimacy in your relationship. Use the following words as your guide, and say them to each other. See who can come up with more words that heighten all of the five senses. The winner gets to be the receiver of pleasure.

Touch

Breasts, thighs, lower back, neck, nipples, eye lids, cheeks, lips, knees, fingertips, sheets, ice cubes, lotion, oil, vulva, vagina, penis, testicles, perineum, scrotum, anus, feathers, brush, comb, flogger, whip, handcuffs, pillows, blankets, towels, metal, cushions, lace, satin, sand, water, mouth, tongue, bubbles, belly button, hair, fabric, wall, bed.

Smell

Candles, sweat, perfume, ocean, autumn leaves, spring air, massage oil, incense, scented lubricant, chocolate, champagne, beer, wine, fresh sheets, lavender, cinnamon rolls, musk, forest, evergreens, caramel, flowers, cut grass, lotion, body butter, hand cream, candy, cologne, spices, gum, firewood, charcoal, berries, citrus, suntan lotion, aloe, vanilla, breath, mint, cookies, lavender, jasmine, orange blossom, oregano, eucalyptus.

Sight

Hot bodies bumping, thrusting, muscles, stomach, bouncing breasts, buttocks, eyes, sweat dripping, hard penis, erect nipples, peach fuzz, open mouth, penetration, lubrication, arched back, mirror image, pornography, open window, video camera, skin, lingerie, blindfold, orgasmic expression, smile, ejaculation.

If you leave out one of the five senses when making love, then you are missing out on 20 percent of pleasure.

Taste

Pussy, semen, tongue, alcohol, peanut butter, salt, honey, chocolate, mint, flavored lubes, vanilla, syrup, skin, sweat, mouthwash, whipped cream, latex, candy, dildo, penis, pre-cum, tears, lip gloss, fingers, water, strawberries, cherries, gum, toothpaste, juice, wine, pizza, cinnamon, celery.

Sound

Moaning, deep breathing, screaming, panting, sighing, heart pounding, music, birds chirping, rustling in the sheets, squeaking bed, banging head board, people pounding that it's too loud, traffic, skin slapping, laughing, giggling, growling, howling, purring, sniffling, weeping, bed springs, humidifier, fan, furnace, wood crackling, vibrator, curtains blowing, spanking, balls slapping, lover's voice, running water.

Sexy Word Games

A few sexy words can turn a boring night into something hot and heavy, and that's exactly how these games are played and won.

Romance in a Jar

Write down all of your romantic wishes, put them in a jar, and give them to your lover to read out loud. Then make a promise to each other to make at least three of them come true.

Cuddle Talk

After making love, cuddle your lover and give him or her verbal action replay of how great the sex was. Be sure to tell it in graphic detail.

Cuddling is also a great time to talk to your lover about future sex activities that you would like to try, such as new sex games.

A Love Puzzle

Buy a small jigsaw puzzle and put it together. Then turn it over and write a sexy message on the back of the whole puzzle. Take it apart and let your partner know that there is a special message, or request, waiting for him or her on the back of the puzzle. See how quickly they can put it together.

Finger Licking Good

Take turns at writing messages with your finger or tongue on each other's body, guess what's being written and see who gets in the last word.

Lust Songs

Make up a song for your partner to let him or her know what's on your mind. For example, "I'm going to ravage you tonight yeah." Ask them to respond back to you in song. For example, "Not until you tease me, kiss me, lick me, oooh."

Wish List Exchange

If you were granted three wishes for your lover to perform, what would they be? Write them down, exchange them, and read them out loud to each other. Make one come true immediately, the next within a week, and the third within a month.

How You Like It

Just like telling a waiter how you want your steak cooked, tell your lover how you want your loving—romantic, passionate, playful, dominating, submissive, experimental, wild, or any other way that turns you on.

Romantic Word Scrabble

Play Scrabble using only words that are romantic and sexy. If you are questioned about a word you use, prove its romantic or sexy value by using it in a sentence. That part alone is half the fun.

Some words you can use in your Scrabble game are throb, pump, caress, rub, quiver, thrust, blow, massage, lube, lick, kiss, suck, stroke, squeeze, fondle, spread, hump, and lust.

Sexy Alphabet Game

One person starts with a letter A and has to do something sensual on their partner's body part that begins with that letter. For example, put his "ankle" between your breasts or tickle the inside of her "arm" with your tongue. Then the other person starts with the letter B and so on and so on.

Sex Boggle

Using the game of Boggle, shake the container with the letter dice and come up with only words that are sexual such as sexy, hot, wet, hard, deep, wild, horny, juicy, lips, stud, and cock.

Finish This Sentence

With answers relating to sex, you and your partner have to finish saying these five sentences at the same time. Be sure to act out the ones you share.

1. You didn't know I ...

2. I wish you would ...

3. I love it when you ...

4. I wish we could ...

5. I won't ...

Story Time

Tell each other sexy bedtime stories by reading erotica from classics like, *Lady Chatterley's Lover* or *The Story of O*. If more modern literature is more your style, try reading, *Deep Inside: Extreme Erotic Fantasies; Frenzy: 60 Stories of Sudden Sex;* or *Enchanted: Erotic Bedtime Stories for Women*.

Checkered Out

Play checkers and any time you move a piece, make a sexy sound, like moan or groan. If you jump one of your partner's pieces, become more verbal, saying "Oh yea!" If you get a king, be more explicit, like "Baby, you feel so good!" This could be the hottest game of checkers you've ever played.

Dirty Talk Games

These dirty talk games can lead to the hottest, wildest, most gratifying sex you've ever had. If you can think it, then you can, and should, say it.

Penis Vagina Talk

Face your partner completely naked with legs apart and imagine if your vagina or penis could talk and tell your lover everything it wanted, what would it say? For example:

1. I love to be licked.

2. What about my balls?

3. I like it when you're gentle.

4. It turns me on when you make the first move.

5. I want to cum first.

Truth or Dare

In this classic game, plan your questions carefully so that you will have the kind of sex you desire. For example, "I dare you to masturbate in front of me until you cum." Or, "Tell me the truth; would you ever go to a swing club?"

Erotic Compliments

Give each other sexual compliments during lovemaking. Tell your partner that he has the most beautiful penis in the world or she has the prettiest pussy ever.

Name Those Genitals

Naming each other's private parts can be fun and very sexy. You can use famous couples like Napoleon and Josephine, Cleopatra and Caesar, Bonnie and Clyde, Tom and Jerry, Thelma and Louise, or make up your own nicknames.

By naming your genitals, you can talk about them in public and nobody will know what you're talking about, but the two of you. For example, "Cleo is feeling neglected, so let's bury Caesar tonight."

Erotic Questions to Ask Him

Whisper these questions in his ear and make sure he answers you word for word, not just with a "Yes." Tell him that you will only do it, if he asks for it.

1. Do you want me to suck your cock until you cum?

2. Do you want me to lick your balls while you rub your cock?

3. Do you want me to sit on your cock and fuck you?

His Erotic Fill-Ins

Tell him to fill in the blanks and then you will fulfill his desires.

1. _____ me.

2. It feels so good when you touch my _____.

3. I want you to _____ my _____.

Erotic Questions to Ask Her

Give her three questions that she must answer back word for word, such as:

1. Do you want me to lick your pussy?

2. Do you want to suck my cock while I lick your pussy?

3. Do you want me to fuck your pussy?

Her Erotic Fill-Ins

Tell her to fill in the blanks and then you will fulfill her desires.

1. _____ me in the _____.

2. It makes me cum when you _____.

3. I love it when you _____ me.

10 Days of Sex

Write down your top 10 favorite sex activities in order of arousal and exchange the list with your lover. For example: kissing, receiving oral sex, mutual masturbation, using sex toys, quickies, role-playing, watching porn, missionary position, 69, anal. Choose one activity from each other's list to do each day for 10 days.

Phone Sex

Talking dirty on the phone can be fun and naughty whether your partner is far away or in the next room. Here are some exciting phone sex games, so wet your lips, lose your inhibitions, and get ready to have sizzling hot phone sex.

Undressing

Make a phone sex date. Then start your phone sex game by asking each other what you are wearing. Then describe taking off each piece of clothing step-by-step.

Let Your Fingers Do the Talking

Start masturbating and describe to each other where you are touching yourself with graphic details. Be sure to moan with pleasure while your lover is narrating his or her masturbation.

Hot Body Talk

Take turns giving each other compliments using long erotic sentences to describe your lover's body. For example "Your sexy, smooth, silky, skin on the inside of your thighs is so delicate to my touch and your perfectly pretty pussy tastes so sweet and delicious." The winner is never at a loss for words.

Hang On, Don't Hang Up

Keep talking erotically on the phone to get your lover to climax before you do. Let each other know what talk is really doing the trick.

Listen In

If you can't be with your lover and don't want them to miss out on your solo fun, have no fear. Simply call your partner, set your phone on the bed, and let them listen to you masturbate. For your partner, the sounds of hearing you rub yourself and/or use a vibrator while moaning and climaxing can be highly erotic.

When Oral Calls

If your partner is on the phone with someone else and continues to be distracted, make him or her squirm with delight by going down on him or her during the call. As long as it's not a really important call, he or she will love the distraction.

Sex Talk Fantasies

Sharing sex fantasies is a fun way to open your relationship up to new activities and can turn predictable sex into exciting adult play.

Set the Scene

Begin a fantasy by creating your wildest scenario and then let your lover add on to it. For example, "I'm getting turned on watching you undress another guy/girl. You look so hot as you go down on him/her." Take turns creating the additional scenes.

Set the Scene is also fun with groups of people who can keep the fantasy going for as many people as there are in the group.

Fantasy Cards

Write down all the fantasies you can both think of on blank cards and then put them into two piles. The first pile should be for fantasies that you both want to turn into reality. The second pile for fantasies that should just remain as fantasies.

Fantasy Places

Describe a place where you would like to have an erotic adventure by giving your partner clues and see how long it takes him or her to guess. Perhaps it's that you want to make out or have sex at a concert, a vineyard, a hotel, on an airplane, in a garden, on a cruise, in a furniture store, at your parents' house, or in an amusement park. All correct guesses get to be acted out.

Techno Sex Games

Describing your sexual desires by "sexting" (texting) explicit messages to your lover can jump-start your sex drive and cause you to climax quickly when you're finally together with him or her.

The Bare Facts

Exchange explicit photos before you have sex with someone new. This can take a lot of pressure off when you already know what the other person looks like, and it can build your sexual energy and desire.

Sending nude photos via cell phone can end up being revealed to the world, so be very careful who you are sexting them to.

Sexting Teaser

Send each other some of these common acronyms to see if your partner knows what they are and responds with more sexting messages to tease you back with.

1. DUSL: Do You Scream Loud?

2. IF/IB: In the Front or In the Back?

3. SorG: Straight or Gay

4. ILF/MD: I Love Female/Male Dominance

5. DUM: Do You Masturbate?

The Vibrating Man/Woman

Set your phone to the VIBRATING setting. For ladies, set your phone on top of your clitoris, and for guys you can set your phone on your perineum or frenulum. Then send your partner texts to elicit a sweet surprise while they watch or read erotica.

Web Caming

Just like phone sex, but with the added visuals, web caming is a great way to add variety to your sex life and get each other off. See who can reach their orgasm first by masturbating and talking dirty to each other.

4

Kissing Games

A kiss can be one of the most romantic, sensual, and erotic exchanges, on a first date or in a lasting relationship. With so many different types and ways of kissing, kisses make for a great playing field for lovers to have fun, get close, or go wild.

In this chapter, you'll discover lots of different kinds of kissing games guaranteed to add more fun and spontaneity to your love life.

Kissing Connections

Kisses initiate and lead the way to a wide spectrum of sexual sensations and connections, from deep and soulful to fun and playful to wild and crazy. Play with these different kinds of kisses and explore the different worlds they can open to you and your partner.

Spiritual

The Eye-Gazer

Tilting your head will help you to maintain eye contact with your partner as you move in for this intimate kiss. At first contact, part your lips slightly and cup your partner's face with one hand. Continue to look into each other's eyes as you open your mouth wider and circle the tip of your tongue around your lover's tongue.

The Tantric Kiss

Begin by placing your prominent hand on each other's heart and then barely touch lips to feel the energy flow between your heart and lips uniting the two of you on a higher level of consciousness. Begin your kiss tenderly in slow motion, opening your mouths for a deeper more intense kiss as you feel each others heart's beating.

The Breather

Synchronize your breathing with your partner by blowing into each other's mouths gently at the same time with lips touching. You are sharing your life force energy, which can lead to a mind, body, and spirit breath connection.

Saucy

The Tease

Begin by using your tongue to trace around your partner's lips and then spread them apart with your tongue. With open mouths, lips not quite touching, flick your tongues against each other teasingly and don't be surprised if this fun kiss makes you want to giggle.

The Nipper

Clasp your lips together over your partner's top lip and then start nipping in short fast motions. Repeat the same motion with their bottom lip. There is no tongue or teeth in this romantic playful kiss.

The Hot Furnace

Sip your favorite hot beverage and let the liquid heat up your mouth before you give your partner a passionate lingering kiss.

Wet

The French Kiss

This super wet kiss can lead to a steamy make-out session as you gradually open your lips; so one of your lips is sandwiched between your partner's. Continue lip locking until you are ready to touch tongue to tongue. Then flick your tongue over theirs, while moving your lips in a slow circular motion together.

A **Make-Out Kiss** is a continuation of the **French Kiss,** following the same steps, but with strong passionate movements including your hands and legs wrapped around each other creating an unforgettable kissing experience.

The Tingler

Put a mint in your mouth while French kissing and pass it back and forth between your mouths to give you both a tingly sensation.

Seductive

Lip-o-Suction

There's no tongue, but plenty of lip-o-sucking of your partner's top and bottom lips very gently. The trick is for you and your partner to kiss the opposite lips so that while you're sucking their bottom lip, they are sucking your top lip.

The Sipper

Take a sip of your favorite drink, whether it's orange juice, wine, champagne, or tasty liquor and deliberately leave a droplet on your lips so that your partner can gently suck the liquid off, then move into a full body *Make-Out Kiss*.

Hard

The Vacu-Sucker

This is a passionate wide-mouthed kiss where both of your lips are completely sealed together before you start sucking air out of your partner's mouth.

The Vampire

Be sure to get your lover's permission before you give a Vampire kiss because, much like a hickey, it will leave a mark. Then kiss him or her on the neck using your mouth like a vacuum, sucking at the skin for about 30 seconds. The intense suction creates a circular purplish bruise proving that they have been taken.

The Primitive Kiss

Take control like a caveman or cavewoman by catching your partner and pulling their hair as you plant a big wet passionate kiss on their lips.

If hair pulling is too rough for your partner, run your fingers through their hair instead and give them a Primitive Kiss.

Sexy

The Fruity Kiss

Take a small piece of fruit such as a strawberry, piece of melon, pineapple, or mango and place it between your lips. Kiss your partner and nibble one half of the fruit while he or she nibbles the other half, allowing the juice to run into your mouths. Lick and kiss around your partner's mouth and chin to taste every last drop.

The Good-Bye Kiss

As your lover turns to leave for work, pull him or her back for a long, wet French kiss and just before you finish, use your tongue to tickle the roof of your partner's mouth. This is a kiss to remember that will make them want to return as soon as they can.

The Orgasmic Kiss

This is especially erotic for men because they have a *frenulum* under the tongue as well as one under the head of the penis. For an orgasmic kissing experience, wiggle your tongue under his tongue to stimulate his frenulum and stimulate his other frenulum down below with your hand.

The **frenulum** is a small fold of tissue that prevents the tongue from moving too far. Whereas the frenulum under the head of the penis connects to the foreskin and is also known as the Sweet Spot for its distinct pleasure.

Deep

The Tongue Sucker

Begin with a slow wet open-mouthed kiss and then wrap your lips around your partner's tongue sucking on it deeply, moving your head back and forth as you increase the speed and intensity of this erotic kiss.

The Chiller

Put an ice cube in your mouth while French kissing and pass it back and forth between your mouths until it melts. This is intensely erotic on a hot day or night.

Quick

The Icy Hot Kiss

One of you drinks something hot while the other drinks something icy cold. You kiss and let your tongues melt each other.

The Lizard

Lock lips and start flicking your tongue in and out of your partner's mouth just like a lizard with short quick strokes. This can be a playful way to greet your partner and help them to forget about a tough day at work.

Kissing Games

Make a break from the same predictable peck on the lips by adding some grown-up playtime into your kissing repertoire. These kissing games will add variety and spice up the lip action of you and your partner.

Make a Bet

Challenge your partner to a kissing contest to determine who can come up with the most different kinds of kisses. (You'll already be ahead if you've read the beginning of this chapter!) The winner gets to make a wish to fulfill a romantic, sensual, or sexual fantasy.

Fingers for Kisses

Take turns giving each other your fingers and choosing different kisses for each finger. For example: Pointer = French Kiss, Ring finger = Make-Out Kiss, Middle finger = Lizard Kiss, Pinky = Tantric Kiss, Thumb = Nip Kiss.

You can play the same game with your toes for kissing, too.

Kiss List

Make a list with two columns of six, with the first column as different kinds of kisses and the second column as different kinds of erogenous body spots. Trade lists with each other and take turns rolling dice and giving and receiving the kiss on the body part that the dice numbers show.

Prisoner of Kisses

With your partner's consent, tie their wrists and blindfold them with scarves. Then kiss him or her where and how you want. You'll be less inhibited because they can't see you and they'll be more excited by the anticipation of not knowing where and how you are going to kiss them.

Kissing Dice

Take two regular dice and assign 12 different types of kisses for each possible number rolled. Make your own rules for the numbers, for instance snake eyes gets a double kiss, rolling a seven chooses any location, and so on.

Oscar Winning Kiss

Pretend that you are the writer, director, and star of a hot steamy movie and your partner is your co-star. Give him or her a kissing scene to perform on you.

If you really want to make your Oscar Winning Kiss authentic, video tape the scene and watch it back together.

On Screen Kiss

Reenact your favorite kissing scenes from movies with your partner. Whether it's from *Pirates of the Caribbean, Closer, Twilight, The Notebook, Mulholland Drive,* or *A Single Man,* this could be the perfect way to create a kissing sensation that surpasses your expectations.

Candy Bar Kiss

Share your favorite candy bar with your date, be it a Hershey Bar, Baby Ruth, Snickers, Kit Kat, or some other favorite candy bar by taking a bite of it and then kissing your partner slowly so that you both experience the same tasty treat. Let your partner know that they get to choose the dessert next time.

Kissing Cards

You'll need the 13 heart cards from a standard deck of playing cards. Have your partner draw a card and give him or her the same amount of kisses as the hearts on the card. Be sure they reciprocate.

Public Display

This is a game lots of adults like to play because there is a thrill in being watched. Arrange to meet at various public places like the shopping mall, at a bar or restaurant, in an elevator, bus stop, or at the airport and kiss your favorite kiss, and see how many different locations you can kiss each other in one day, one week, and one month.

Unlike Public Kissing, *Surprise Kisses* are unexpected and can be in or out of public places. See who can surprise the other the most with kisses while sleeping, showering, working, cooking, shopping, swimming, talking on the phone, riding the bus or train, walking, washing the car, playing golf, or any time of the day or night.

Candyland

Choose two different distinct flavored candies for you and your partner to place on your tongues, such as a cinnamon candy and a mint, lemon drop and butterscotch, coffee and licorice. Then touch lips and try to take each other's candy using only your tongue and mouth.

Lip Smackers

Try on different flavored lip glosses and find one you and your partner like then kiss while wearing the lip gloss. Lip Smackers has a wide variety of flavors like strawberry banana, cotton candy, bubble gum, vanilla, and cherry that can surely entertain your tongue. You can also try on the different flavors and have your partner guess which one it is.

Feel the Vibes

One person places a Screaming O Vibrating Tongue Ring, called The LING-O, on their tongue while they stick it out and gently flick their partner's tongue. Be prepared for some quivering senses.

Catch Me if You Can

Both partners sit face-to-face, one as the instigator and the other is the catcher. The instigator sticks their tongue out while the catcher tries to touch their partner's tongue with their own tongue. If caught, that's one point. The first to three points loses and owes their partner a steamy favor at their request.

Lady and the Tramp

Make spaghetti dinner even more fun by taking a long piece of cooked pasta and putting one end into each other's mouth. Eat your way to the middle and meet for a lingering kiss.

You can use any kind of food that will reach from one mouth to the other, such as a breadstick, piece of asparagus or celery stick, licorice or even a sausage.

Go, Baby, Go Kiss

Set a timer for 30 seconds and see how many dry baby kisses you can plant around your partners face.

Paper-Rock-Scissors

Play the traditional game tapping fists in your palm two times and on the third time choose your rock, paper, or scissors with the appropriate hand gestures. Rock beats scissors and chooses any kind of kiss desired. Scissors beats paper and winner chooses any place to be kissed. Paper beats rock and winner chooses the kind of kiss and place to be kissed.

Secret Kiss Word

Before you go out with your partner to a party, choose a code word. Whenever anyone says that word, you must kiss, so make it a common word such as "Hi" or "You."

Tongue Ring Fun

If your partner has a tongue ring, flick it with your tongue while French kissing to add extra stimulation for him or her. If you both have tongue rings, have a tongue ring battle to see who can keep kissing the longest. Be careful not to chip any teeth. For those of you who do not have a tongue ring, but would like to emulate the sensation of having one, try a magnetic tongue ring that uses suction to stay on.

Kissing with braces can give you the same kinds of erotic sensations as kissing with a tongue ring. Just avoid pushing your lips together too hard and keep your movements slow and sensual.

Animal Kingdom

Get into an animal pose and start acting and kissing your partner until he or she guesses what animal you are. For example, you can nuzzle like a cat, lick like a dog, slither like a snake, or monkey around like an ape.

Group Kissing Games

If you want to add some adult fun to a party, these kissing games (some of which you'll remember from way back when) will create a playful atmosphere, and may result in some unexpected hookups!

Spin the Bottle

This game requires any kind of empty bottle and a group of friends. Sitting in a circle around the bottle, the first person to go spins it and has to kiss whoever the bottle is pointing at when it stops spinning. To up the stakes, choose an area to be kissed before you spin such as the fingers, toes, belly button, and so on.

Suck and Blow

Standing in a circle, one person starts by placing a small square piece of paper to their mouth and holding it there by sucking in with all their might. They turn to the person next to them who has to retrieve the paper by sucking it. When they begin sucking it from the paper holder's lips, the holder blows it to their lips for a smooth transition. If the paper slips, you wind up in a kiss.

7 Minutes in Heaven

Place pieces of paper with the names of people in two different bowls, one for males and one for females. Select from whichever bowl preferred and read the name on the paper. Have the person who selected and the person chosen go into a closet to kiss each other for the next seven minutes.

Unlike 7 Minutes in Heaven, *60 Seconds in Heaven* is where one person wears bright red lipstick and goes into the closet with their selected partner and plants as many kisses on them as they can in 60 seconds. When they come out, the lipstick kisses are counted and the partners with the most kisses are the winners.

Kissing Contest

The couple that can kiss for the longest time is the winner. Be sure to have a sexy gift for them, such as a vibrating sex toy or edible panties.

Copy Kiss

This can be played with as many couples as you want, but the first couple must kiss in a specific position and style and after they have finished, the next couple must copy their exact kissing techniques. This is hilarious to videotape and playback.

Kiss Tag

One person is chosen to be "It" while everyone else runs after him or her. The first one to tag "It" gets to kiss them.

Blind Kiss

One person is blindfolded and must sit on a chair or sofa while everyone takes turns kissing him or her. The blind kisser must guess who is who, based only on the way that they kiss, no touching.

Kisses in the Dark

Turn all the lights off so that everyone is standing in a dark room. Then tell everyone to walk around and when they bump into someone, they have to kiss them.

You might be surprised at who you enjoy kissing in the dark, so be nice to everyone when the lights are turned on!

Have fun!

5

Erotic Massage and Happy Ending Games

In this chapter, your hands and body are going to do the talking as you explore the pleasures of erotic massage games and happy endings that will have you and your lover begging for more.

Begin by setting the mood with candles, soft music, and warming the room, as you are both going to be naked. Pick up some massage oil and lube and you're ready to arouse and evoke sexual intimacy with a memorable erotic massage.

Erotic Body Landmarks

Are you feeling adventurous? Then you may have what it takes to be a body explorer and conquistador of pleasure. Discovering and finding erotic body "landmarks" or pleasure spots on your lover is both a skill and an art form.

Learn these landmarks and how to "play" with them. Ask your lover to rate his or her body landmarks from 1 to 10 on a pleasure scale, with 10 being the best. Be sure to memorize the ones that are eight and above.

The Crown

Some lucky men and women can orgasm from getting a good head massage. They may not know that it's called an extragenital orgasm, but they do know they can't get enough head rubbing, scalp scratching, and hair brushing. Have your lover lay back while you explore their head and hair to bring them pleasure and delight. Also, washing your lover's hair is another sexy way to massage the head.

The Third Eye

The forehead area between the eyebrows is also called the third eye. Tension can build up there and some gentle thumb pressing can release it, so that you feel aroused instead of stressed. With your other hand, let it roam to your lover's heart area and caress gently.

The Eargasm

It's possible to give someone an eargasm when you massage their lobes between your thumbs and fingers. Licking along the outer edge of the ear followed by your warm breath may result in multiple eargasms.

Be a pal and give your partner an eargasm after they perform oral sex on you. What better gift is there than giving a release after getting one?

Neck Tease

Tease your partner by stroking your hands gently up and down, around the front and the back of the neck and end by gently brushing your fingertips to give them shivers of pleasure.

Nipple Tickle

Use your hair to caress the breasts or chest and then use your thumb and index finger to gently massage the nipple in a rotating motion moving clockwise then counterclockwise.

Tummy Touches

A tummy touch tends to tickle, so play nice. Rub plenty of massage oil in your hands and then put your hands lightly on top of the belly button pushing the palm of your hand down in slow circular motions.

Knockin' on Heaven's Door

On her, a heavenly landmark is the region below the stomach where the mons or pubic hair is located above the genitals. Like petting a cat, use your hands to brush the peach fuzz on the softest parts of the skin. If cats love the feeling, so will your partner.

Did you know that the pubic region is loaded with sensitive nerve endings just dying to be massaged? For some women, it's the second most sensitive area of their vulva behind the clitoris. With that kind of info, don't forget to knock on heaven's door more often.

Thigh Land

Let your light, tickly strokes and caresses create sensual anticipation for your lover as you slide your hands up, down, and around the inner and outer thighs.

Back Slide

Place your hands on your lover's lower back and let your hands glide up your lover's back all the way up to the neck, around the shoulders, and all the way down and over the butt.

Bottoms Up

If you've ever kneaded pizza or bread dough, then this technique will be a breeze. But if you haven't, try squeezing your partner's butt between your thumb and fingers in a flowing motion. Then gently spread the cheeks before you move on to the anus, also known as the Rosebud.

The Rosebud

Gently massage the anal ring with light circular strokes. Press on the anal ring with your thumb and ask your lover if he or she would like you to go deeper. If the answer is no, then just continue to massage around the butt cheeks. If the answer is yes, then move your forefinger inward gently paying close attention to your lover's resistance.

As your finger progresses deeper in a man, search for a nut-sized spongy area, which is his prostate gland (the male equivalent of the G-spot), by bending your finger in a "come here" gesture, about two inches inside the Rosebud.

Penetration of the Rosebud can be equally as pleasurable for women. When stimulating the Rosebud, let the receiver be in control and use plenty of lubricant.

Toe Fu

Rotate every toe clockwise and counterclockwise and finally slither your forefinger or tongue between each toe.

Female Flower

Use a water-based lubricant instead of oil to massage the vulva and vagina, gently using the pad of your thumbs to trace the outline of the outer and inner lips.

Clitoral Magic

Gently pull the clitoral hood back from the clitoris to expose it. Then slide your thumb and forefinger up and down the sides of the clitoris for about ten strokes. Massage the head of the clitoris in circular motions using your forefinger.

Male Stalk

Place one hand on the shaft of his penis and start stroking it in an up and down motion while the other hand gently encircles his testicles.

His Million Dollar Point

If you slide your fingers up and down the perineum from his anus to his testicles, you'll feel a small indentation the size of a pea midway known as the Million Dollar Point. Using the pad of your thumb press firmly until your lover asks you to stop or has a climax.

Massage Games

If you want to spend the night with your hands all over each other, then these massage games will quench your sexual appetite. You'll also have the best sex of your life while being playful and intimate.

A Head Scratcher

Purchase a crossword puzzle book and take turns seeing who can guess the most words. Use your mind to win a little head— that's a head massage. With all that brainpower being used, you both deserve it.

A Military Facial

Get your fingers loose and ready for a winner's facial massage as you duke it out over the classic strategy game Battleship. The winner gets a much deserved third eye massage.

Singing Sweethearts

Have a contest with your lover and sing to each other. The person who sings the best receives a sensual eargasm massage by the loser.

To spice up your ear massage, consider giving your hands and fingers a break and use your tongue with a sensual mix of warm breath and moaning. This will surely take your ear massage to the next level.

Lawn Wars

Spend some time outdoors on the lawn together and challenge your partner to a game of catch. The first to drop the ball is the loser and must give the winner a neck tease massage.

Marble Mayhem

Remember playing marbles as a youngster? There's no rule that says we can't enjoy that game again in adulthood. Play a game of marbles with your partner and see who's King or Queen of this hill. The winner gets a genital massage.

For a genital massage, rub his penis with both hands as if rubbing a stick to make a fire. This is a sure way to light his fire! Or for women gently pull the clitoral hood back from the clitoris to expose it and massage with your forefinger.

X's and O's

XO may normally mean hugs and kisses, but for this game it's Tic Tac Toe. Play best of five games with your partner and the winner gets a tummy massage.

Nipples and Dots

Access your creative side and play connect the dots with your lover. Take a piece of paper and draw multiple dots on it. Then copy the paper and let the games begin. The winner is the person who creates the most sexual drawing from the dots. The loser must give their partner a butt massage and play with their dots.

Crazy 8's

Use a deck of cards and separate all the eights, Kings, and Queens. Shuffle these separated cards and lay them flat on your table or bed. Each of you will choose one card and take turns. Each time a person chooses an eight, the other person must massage their lover's toes for 30 seconds. Kings and Queens represent wild cards that allow you to choose how and where you want to be massaged for 30 seconds. Kings mean you choose and Queens mean the opponent chooses. Continue playing until either all four Kings or all four Queens are chosen. Whoever draws the most face cards is the winner and gets a 10-minute back massage with the oil or lotion of their choice.

Jacks or Jill

Play a classic game of jacks against your partner to see who is the champion jacks player in your relationship. The winner earns a full frontal massage while the loser gets to go back to the drawing board and practice their jack skills. Who has the better hand-eye coordination to win this challenge?

Mini Wrestling

Pin your partner's thumbs in this timeless competitive game. Lock hands and try to pin your partner's thumbs underneath your thumb for three seconds. Think you've got the strength for a thumb war? Play best of five and the loser must give the winner a hand massage.

Snakes and Ladders

Relive your childhood play dates with your partner and play a game of Shoots and Ladders. The winner earns their choice of giving or receiving a snakes and ladder massage.

Give your lover a snakes and ladders massage by climbing up an imaginary ladder with your fingertips and slithering like a snake using your tongue on your lover's spine. That should send shivers up and down their body.

Hula Hoop Away

Challenge your partner to a best-of-three hula hoop showdown to see who has more sway to the hips and shake in their bake. Use a timer or watch to see who can last longest keeping a hula hoop going around their waist. The first match the hulas go clockwise, the second is counterclockwise, and the tiebreaker is the direction of your choice. The winner gets a well-deserved clitoral or testes massage.

Pin the Tail on the Booty

Instead of a donkey, use your partner's backside for this sexy game of blindfolded fun. Take two stickers and place one of them on your partner's butt. Spin your partner around three times and have them place the second sticker as close as they can to the other sticker. Take turns and the person that's closest to pinning their tail on the booty receives a butt or million dollar point massage.

For an added bonus, play Pin the Tail on other parts of the body like your nipples or navel. Change up the location of the massage to make the prize new, fresh, and unpredictable.

My Sore Hamstrings

Play Connect 4 with your partner and see who has what it takes to earn a thigh massage. Play best of five and winner gets their legs pampered. Make sure your partner massages both legs.

Candy-Flavored Feet

Break out the Candyland game you have hidden in the closet for a little adult game time. Because the game is focused on walking through different lands, the winner of the game earns a foot massage to pamper their toes from the long travels through candy cane forests and gum drop mountains.

Pass Go and Collect an FBM

What's an FBM you ask? It stands for full body massage. That's right, from head to toe and everything in between. Challenge your partner to a game of Monopoly, with the loser (or the quitter) giving the other person a full body massage for at least 30 minutes.

Synchronized Erotic Massage Games

Some erotic massages can be done simultaneously for his and her pleasure. And why not, it's like hitting two bulls' eyes with one shot. Can you and your lover master the art of mutual massage?

Tantric Body Touch

Have one partner lube himself or herself up with lotion or oil and use their own body to massage their partner. Be creative as a knee, breasts, an elbow, your butt, and even your nose can all be used against your partner's body.

Try using your chin for an added twist during your tantric body touch massage. Have your partner lie on their front and use your chin on the sides of their spine and around the shoulders. For an added bonus, try using small amounts of warming/cooling lube and blow your breath onto the skin as you pass down the back.

Your "O" Face

Try lying side-by-side and facing each other to get a good angle. On him, use both hands in opposite directions in a corkscrew motion over the penis. On her, gently part her outer lips with both of your thumbs and caress them in circular motions. Don't focus on the hands, but on your partner's face as you bring them to their "O" face.

A Privates Massage

Get your genitals and inner thighs lubed up and straddle your partner for a massage from your privates. It will take a bit of hip gyrations and thigh squeezing to create a memorable and original massage. The winner is the person who can bring his or her partner to orgasm the quickest.

Chest Bump

Give your partner a breast or chest massage with your lubed up genitals. Ride your partner and give them a massage they'll never forget. You are sure to enjoy it, too.

Lending a Hand

Take turns masturbating in front of your partner with an added twist; place your hand on your partner's hand as they touch themselves. You'll get to feel their motions, learn their masturbatory style, which will hopefully translate into giving better genital massages.

Masturbate-a-thon

Have a mutual masturbation-a-thon and set aside an entire evening to focus on each other's genitals. For him, massage the penis from the top to the bottom covering the head and sliding your hands down to the base with one hand after another in a fluid motion. For her, rub the clitoris with one hand and insert a finger into the vagina with the other.

Scissor-cise

Lube up your genitals and interlock your legs together for a yoga pose you'll never forget. Grind your genitals into your partner's genitals as you gaze into each other's eyes. The energy of joining your two genitals should send sparks throughout.

Happy Ending Games for Him

Massage parlors may have made happy endings famous, but your new skills are going to make you a legend and keep him coming back for more. A little oil and lube goes a long way in the pleasure department, so stock up like the erotic massage pros do and get ready for a few different strokes for horny folks.

The Healing Stroke

Make a bet about the weather outside and if he's close to correct, then raise his temperature by giving him this happy ending–healing stroke massage. Using your palm rub down the underbelly of his shaft to the testes and back up the shaft to the head. Keep going up and down and you'll see that these long strokes have a healing power on him.

Praying Mantis

Ask him to tell you your favorite sex position and if he's right, place your hands together as if you were clapping. Put his penis snuggly inside your clasped palms. Now slide your hands in opposite directions while keeping them together. The fingertips and the opposite hand palm will end up touching and become lined up. Continue doing this motion and incorporate an up and down direction on the shaft. He'll be praying for more in no time.

Fire Starter

Tell him to guess your bra size and if he gets it right, place the shaft of his penis in your hands and begin to move your hands in forward and backward motion. It will look as if you were trying to start a fire or warm up your hands with his penis.

Don't forget to focus on the head of his penis and his frenulum, which is located where the head and shaft meet on the under belly of the penis. Most men squirm with pleasure when these areas are stroked.

Twist and Shout

Ask him to describe where to find your G-spot. If it sounds good, then grip his penis shaft with one hand twisting it in a corkscrew motion up and down. With your other hand, place your palm on the head of his penis and rub in circular motions.

The Barbershop Corkscrew

Ask him to name three of your erotic body landmarks. If he can, then use both hands to grip his penis and twist in a corkscrew motion in opposite directions. He won't know what hit him. Add an up and down motion to really get him twitching to orgasm.

Double Trouble

Ask him if he knows what your favorite aphrodisiac is. If he answers correctly, use lots of lube to get him nice and slippery from his testes up to his penis. With one hand, masturbate his penis in an up and down corkscrew motion. With the other hand, massage his testes and give him a double dose of pleasure.

Triple Threat

Tell him to kiss you for two minutes or longer. If he does, then reward him by rubbing his anus and perineum with long strokes. With the other hand, do the healing stroke where you stroke from testicles to the tip of his penis.

Happy Ending Games for Her

Show her that you know what to do in between her legs and forever reap the benefits of being a good lover. Her happy ending may turn out to be your happy beginning.

The Magic Button

Hide a penny in one hand and tell her to guess which hand it's in. If she chooses the right hand, do your magic trick on her magic button, the clitoris. Get to know the style of clitoral touch she likes from circular motions, side-to-side or up/down, the tempo, speed, and amount of pressure. Don't give up until she has her happy ending.

Palms Away

Get two flashlights and put them on in the dark. Move your spotlight around the room and if your lover can move her light over yours, she wins a happy ending. Use your palm to whisk her away on a pleasure-filled ride by lubing up your palm and covering her entire vulva with it. Move your palm in circular and up and down motions over her mons and vulva and watch her reaction.

Peace, Love, and Happiness

Ask your lover to tell you what your favorite way to orgasm is and if she gets it right, reward her with a happy ending of her own. Lie next to her and lube up her vulva for a happy ending 60's style. Use your index and middle fingers and pleasure her with a peace sign. Start by having your two fingers close together at her clitoris and slide down the sides of her vaginal lips. If you go all the way down her vulva, part of the palm of your hand will also slide by her clitoris.

Thumb Shiatsu

Play "I spy with my little eye" and think of something erotic to make it easy for her to win. While sitting in front of her vulva as she lies on her back, use your two thumbs to give her labia a massage. Try the up/down, side/side, or circular motions to give her different sensations. Then bring one thumb up to the clitoris while the other stays with the labia massage. Rotate occasionally and you'll see how the clitoris and the labia can work in perfect harmony together.

Come Here Baby

Ask your lover to describe how to massage the male prostate. If it sounds good, reward her by massaging her G-spot. Have her lie down on her back. Take one or two fingers and insert them into her love canal. On the upper wall of her vagina, is her G-spot. Motion your fingers as if you were motioning for a person to come to you and witness the power of internal fingering.

The Corkscrew

Ask your lover what kind of animal she thinks that you are in bed. If you like her answer, give her the corkscrew. Insert two fingers and cross them over as if you were crossing your fingers when telling a lie. Next, twist your fingers in a corkscrew motion and watch her go wild with the full, ribbed feeling of your fingers.

Try the windshield wiper with your corkscrew. While you're corkscrew fingering, use your thumb to go past the clitoris in a side-to-side windshield wiper motion to add a little zing.

The Double Decker

Tell her to rub her stomach while tapping her head for 60 seconds. If she does it, give her the ultimate happy ending. Use one hand to massage her mons, clitoris, and vaginal opening in a circular fashion and use the other hand to massage her perineum and anus in an up and down stroke. I promise, it's easier than rubbing your stomach and tapping your head.

6

Games Around the House

You don't have to go out on a date or visit a sex shop to play sex games, as you have everything you need within your reach inside your home. You may just want to stay home more often!

In this chapter, you'll discover how to play sex games in every room in your home and use your household items in ways you never thought possible to add more excitement to your love life.

Steamy Bathroom Games

Heat things up in the bathroom with your lover to turn it into a pleasure palace! You'll never take your bathroom for granted again after playing some of these steamy, sudsy, wet, and wild games with your lover.

Sponge Babe

Before making love, surprise your lover with a sensual sponge bath and explore his or her body. Be creative with scented soaps, such as lavender, almond, or sandalwood. Use perfumed oils to increase your lover's olfactory pleasure. In this game, the receiver must be the giver of a sponge bath after lovemaking.

Blow Job

After bathing together, ask your lover if he or she wants a blow job. When they say, "Yes," use a hair dryer to blow-dry your lover, starting at the toes and working your way up. If you linger in the mid-section, that's understandable, then continue on up their body finishing by drying and styling your lover's hair.

Perfectly Bare

Shaving is a boring task, so make it more enjoyable by shaving your lover's face, legs, armpits or anything else you can make "baby bottom" smooth. A steady hand is required for this game, so whoever can pull out all of the tissues from a tissue box without moving it and using one hand is the shaver.

Don't forget to use mirrors for that extra erotic visual stimulation.

Lovers Slide

Lather each other up in the shower and slide your bodies together like human washcloths and with an egg in between you. The object of the game is not to break the egg, but if you do at least you'll be in the right place to clean up.

If you love having sex in the shower, get your lover the Dual Locking Suction Handle by Sportsheets. It has two lockdown suction areas to help you achieve any position and add instant leverage for better performance.

Water Fight

Place small dabs of toothpaste on your erotic hot spots and have a bet with your lover to see how many he or she can reach using a Water-Pic's pulsating stream of water, or the shower head. Adjust the pressure and direction as indicated by your lover's responses.

Toothbrush Tickle

Have a tickle contest using a new soft-bristle toothbrush as you lightly stroke your lover's body, teasing all those little nooks and crannies. Next time your dentist gives you a complimentary toothbrush, save it for this pleasurable activity.

Sex in the Tub

Ignite your lover's passion by making out on some nice fluffy towels on the floor and then step into the warm water-filled tub to climax. The object of the game is to hold your orgasm back until you get into the bath.

An erotic way to have sex in the shower is to hold onto the shower rod while having sex standing up. Make sure it's firmly attached to the wall first.

Kinky Kitchen

Get ready to turn your kitchen into a palatable palace of pleasure as you cook up hot games of passion adding sizzle and spice to your love life.

Counters and Chairs

One of you sits on the kitchen counter and the other in a kitchen chair. Play paper, rock, scissors and the winner gets to decide who is on the counter to receive oral sex and who is in the chair giving it.

Milk and Cookies

You both put a cookie on your foreheads and try to move the cookie into your mouth without touching it. The winner gets to pour milk on the loser and lick it off.

Sugar and Spice

Have a contest to see who can frost a cake the fastest. The loser has to fill a sifter with powdered sugar and sprinkle it over their lover's body liberally and lick it clean.

Spatula Spanking

Give your lover a little spanking with a spatula or wooden spoon when he or she answers their phone during quality time with you. You'll be pleasantly surprised at how few calls they will be taking, unless they enjoy being spanked.

Straw-Blowing

Use a soda straw to blow gently in his or her ear and watch how your cool breath evokes a pleasurable shudder. Then blow your breath all the way down your lover's neck toward the nipples and keep going south. The game is to see how long it takes your lover to beg you to make love to them.

Don't blow into a woman's vagina since it can be dangerous because excessive air in the blood stream could cause an embolism, but do blow on top of her body for breathless responses.

Icy Hot

Have a marathon to see who can take a freezing wet cloth from the freezer and put it on their hot body the longest. The winner gets to choose any location to have sex.

Icing on the Cake

Fill a cake decorator with icing, or you can fill a small plastic sandwich bag and cut off a corner, and use it to write notes and messages on your lover's body. Add emphasis to the words as you "erase" them with your tongue. Your lover must be able to read the words in order to have his or her orgasm.

Body Basting

Give your lover an erotic massage with a basting brush dipped in some warm oil. Baste your lover's most sensitive areas with the warm, silky brush.

Use the basting brush dipped in warm oil to stroke around your lover's earlobe, up and down the neck, armpit, shoulders, nipples, navel, inside of the thighs, and around the buttocks.

Giant Vibrations

Make doing laundry fun by sitting on top of your tumble dryer while it's drying your clothes and let yourself feel the vibrations ripple through your loins. Better still, tell your lover that you want to be rewarded for your hard work by having sex on top of the tumble dryer for a unique sensation you'll talk about for months to come.

Dust and Tickle

See who can flip the most bottle caps into a cup. The winner gets to have their body teased and titillated with a clean feather duster. To increase the erotic effect, blindfold your lover so they can anticipate where the duster will tickle next.

Bedroom Bliss

Spice up your sex life with these sex games in the bedroom. If you have kids, be sure to lock your door.

The Flasher

Whoever has the most freckles gets to be pampered by their lover. Lie down naked and let your lover count your freckles using a flashlight. Make sure all the lights are off and it's pitch black. Each new freckle must be kissed and then counting continues until both sides of the body have been thoroughly examined and loved.

Boudoir Paparazzi

Bounce pencils into a glass and whoever gets the most into the glass gets to take some sexy boudoir photos of their lover. Start by snapping pictures of your lover fully clothed, then slowly undress and pose. You can get more adventurous as your lover becomes more comfortable in front of the camera.

Sex Alarm

Whoever goes to sleep last must set the alarm clock one hour earlier than usual so you can spend extra time with your lover. Making love in the morning will help to ease the stress of the day and create a bond that lasts till dinner. Make this an unexpected ritual.

Sex-opoly

Take your Monopoly game, or any other board game you have, and sex it up by changing the rules. Monopoly can be sexy when you play naked and if you land on "Go to Jail" then your lover handcuffs you while making love to you.

Sexman

Play the game similar to Hangman, but all of the words must be sexual and the winner gets to have their orgasm first.

A Little Head or Tail

All you need to play this game is a coin and a naughty list to have fun all night long. Make a naughty list of sexy actions like erotic massage and role-playing for the winner to choose from. Just keep flipping the coin and keep choosing from the list.

Sex Cards

Put together a deck of cards by using your own photos, the sexier the better. Shuffle and spread all the cards face down, then take turns flipping them over to see if you can make a matching pair. The player with the most matches wins a sexual favor.

You can also sex up a regular deck of cards by assigning each card a sexual activity and then acting out whatever the card describes.

Heart Hunter

This game is inexpensive, creative, and romantic as you cut hearts out of colored paper and leave them all around your bedroom leading up to where you want to have sex. Be sure to number them and write sexy messages on each one that will motivate your lover to keep on looking for the next heart.

Rec Room Thrills

Sex is adult play, and what better place to play than in the recreation room?

Game of Cards

Using index cards, list different furniture on each card (sofa, ottoman, coffee table, accent table, pool table, end table, chair, recliner, etc.). Shuffle the cards and select one at random. Then, make love any way you want to on that piece of furniture.

Pop It

You'll need to blow up about a dozen balloons for this game and place them in-between your bodies as you hug and kiss, being careful not to pop them. For each balloon that bursts you must do something more intimate to your lover like oral sex, or whatever they want.

Basketball Sex

Set up a small basketball hoop and take turns shooting hoops. With each dunk, the winner gets to choose a kiss or lick in a certain place.

Dirty Pool

If you have a pool table in your home, you'll love this game, which is played the same way as regular pool, except that you must distract your lover from playing his or her shot. The distractions should be sexual like kissing, spanking, or even flashing them. At the end of the game, climb on the table and the winner gets to choose their pleasure.

The X-Rated Box

If your lover is hooked on video games, tell him or her to teach you how to play and then bet sexual favors for the winner.

Naked Football

Play a game of naked football in your rec room. You'll have some idea as to how to score points, especially if he plays quarterback and she plays center.

Living Room Love

Don't let your living room become stuffy where only visitors sit and socialize. Make it a living room for loving with these sexy games.

The Ritual

Start by christening all the furniture in your living room by having sex in different positions on every chair, on the couch, on the floor, the piano, against the bookcase, in front of the TV, and on or below the coffee table (as long as it's safe). You'll have so much fun seeing family and friends sitting or eating at places where you've had sex.

You will become far more attached to your furniture after you and your lover have used it for sex.

Blanket Spread

Spread a blanket on the floor and grease each other up with some aromatherapy massage oil from WET, System JO, or one from your local drug store. Then use your body to massage your lover as you slide from side to side, up and down.

Commercial Sex

This game is played while watching TV with your lover, whether you are both watching sports, a TV series, or even the news. The idea is to make out during each commercial break and then stop as soon as the program resumes. If you're lucky, you won't make it through watching the whole show.

Dining Room Delights

Eating will never be the same at your dining room table with family and friends. These games will create memories you'll never forget.

Three Minutes to Win It

Between the appetizer, main meal, and dessert, make out with your lover for three minutes to win the next course.

Table Dance

Whoever cooked dinner or paid for takeout gets to receive a lap dance and striptease on the dining room table.

Clear the Table

After sharing a tasty, seductive meal and all the dirty dishes are on the table, passionately clear the table sending all the dishes crashing to the floor as you and your lover climb on top of the table for your own version of dessert.

Strip Checkers, Chess, or Backgammon

All of these games are fun to play at the dining room table while dinner is in the oven, especially if you set the scene for a romantic evening with candles and music. The rules are simple: the winner takes off an article of clothing from the loser's body until naked or dinner is ready to be served.

Sex Puzzle

The dining room table is the best place to put together a puzzle, and putting this puzzle together is going to be a unique experience. For every piece you pick up and put in the puzzle, tell your lover something sexual about yourself and/or something you want to do to him or her. See how far you get with the puzzle before you're on the table doing what you've said. It may take you a while to put this puzzle together.

You can also make a sexy puzzle using a revealing photo of yourself that is sure to please your lover. Scan the picture and glue it onto a puzzle or a piece of cardboard, then carefully, cut out the puzzle pieces. Let your lover put it together and see how much they like to do this puzzle.

Outside Fun

Playing outside your home can be even more exhilarating than playing inside no matter what season. Whether it's spring time with birds singing, summer under the scorching sun, autumn in the cool breeze, or winter in the snow or rain, having sex outdoors can bring you closer together, creating fun playful memories.

Naked Camping

Take a tent and go camping in your backyard. Pack a warm sleeping bag. Snuggle up by sharing one bag between you or zip two together. The object of the game is to undress each other while inside the bag. Wake up early and watch the sun (and other things) rise.

Wax On and Turn On

Turn washing the car into a game by doing it together and having a wet T-shirt contest as you throw suds at each other. It may take longer than the local car wash but you'll have fun getting wet while wiping your car clean together.

Once your car is nice and clean on the outside, how about getting dirty on the inside? It may be cramped in the front, so climb in the back to make love. This may take you back to your teenage years.

Sex Tag

Play an old fashioned game of tag. Start outside then move it inside so that the winner initiates having sex in any room they want.

Hula Hoop

Have a hula hoop contest to see who can hula hoop the longest. The winner gets to choose where to make love outside the house after dark.

Slip and Slide

Create a slip and slide with long plastic sheets or large garbage bags and a bottle of baby oil. Grease up your slip and slide and have a contest to see who can slide the farthest with a one-step, two-step, or three-step head start. Play this game in an area that allows for a little mess and provides some cushioning such as on an old mattress or in the back yard on the grass. Enjoy a shower together afterward, too.

Shoot Me

Water guns are perfect for water fights and you can chase each other around to see who can get the other wetter. Ladies, be sure to wear a white flimsy T-shirt and let your lover win.

Hide and Sex

Leave a note on your door for your lover to find when he or she comes home that simply reads, "Find Me." Much like the favorite game of hide and seek, this adult version is just as much fun, especially when the seeker sexually seduces the hider wherever they are hiding. You could be in the car, the garden, the shed, the porch, on the deck, or anywhere outside you'd like to have some sexual fun.

7

Playful Positions and Props

In this chapter, let your body do the talking as you take a walk on the wild side with sexy positions and games with props to bring out the animal in you. Who says making love needs to only be a missionary experience? So stretch out your back and those tight hamstrings because this chapter is going to test not only your mind and imagination, but also your muscles and flexibility.

We'll be working from the basic sex positions—Missionary, Doggy-Style, Cowgirl, Reverse Cowgirl, Spooning, Scissors, and standing positions. We'll also throw in a few curveball positions and games for those who can handle something a bit more advanced.

Oral Sex Positions and Games

Getting into various oral sex positions only adds to the enjoyment, and you'll find that different positions can make you feel different sensations. So have fun with these positions and games and be sure to tell your lover which ones excite you the most.

Licking Her Landscape

The position a woman is in to receive oral sex can be just as important as the licking itself. So get comfortable and try something new, as each position described here will take her in a new direction of pleasure and imagination.

The Explorer

One of the most comfortable and popular positions for a woman to receive oral sex is while lying on her back. To spice it up, wear a low beam headlamp whenever she wants you to go down on her and let her describe graphically how she wants her treasure to be explored.

Lily Pad Licks

Women masturbate to orgasm using this position, and there's no reason why you can't use it for oral sex. Have her lie on her stomach and arch her vulva and buttocks out that gives her "lily pad" a new angle for oral kisses. Have a bet on who can wait the longest before penetration. The winner gets to have another oral orgasm.

The Doggy Lick

Have her get on all fours and reap the amazing benefits of this position. Give her oral sex from behind while she stays on her hands and knees or kneels down.

Some may find the Doggy position a bit difficult to access the clitoris. Have no fear, a pillow or two beneath her pelvis and abdomen will raise her vulva to the perfect spot for your mouth to hum the most perfect orgasm tune.

Power Grind

Let her get on top of your face while you lie down to give her an oral treat you both won't soon forget. Being on top gives her the power to move her hips and grind her vulva onto your lips or tongue. Have a bet to see how long until she climaxes. The winner gets a genital massage.

The Reverse Grind

Take that Power Grind position and flip around, so she is facing your feet. This will give you a bit more clitoral access and a visual of her backside. The game is to see who can talk dirty for the longest. The winner gets to make a fantasy their reality.

If she likes the Grind positions, make sure you have enough space to breathe. Unless smothering you with all her magical goodness is part of the oral thrill you seek.

The Statue of Liberty

Have her stand up and you kneel before her, offering her an oral gift. For her it's quite a powerful position wouldn't you say? See how long she can handle your oral gift.

Licking His Lollipop

One of the most favorite gifts a guy loves to receive is oral sex. So don't get stuck with the same old routine, try some variety to give him the feeling of the first time every time.

The Hammock

Lying on his back, he'll feel like he's in a hammock on a tropical island while receiving oral sex. First, play a game of Limbo to see how low you can go.

The Tortoise

Take a page from our relaxed animal friend and get comfortable in a face down position over him. Extend his penis and lick the underside of the penis from head to scrotum. Count how many licks you give him before he wants intercourse or orgasm.

Puppy Pose

With the enthusiasm of a playful puppy, have your man get on all fours. You can perform oral sex from beneath him and have the freedom to reach him from all angles. Taking the puppy pose a step further, play a naked version of the game Twister. Have him reach each color while in the Doggie-Style position. Once in position, suspend the game and crawl up under him for a round of naked twister fellatio.

The Chariot

He'll feel like a gladiator as he kneels on top of you and receives oral sex. Let the gladiator glide his "sword" across your face, neck, nipples, and any other places he'd like to conquer.

If he craves making love to your face, make sure he's aware of how deep he thrusts and how fast he penetrates. He will reap the rewards in the end.

Push Up

This reverse Chariot position will have his penis inside your mouth while he faces your genitals. Have him do push ups over you while facing your feet, and when you think he's done enough, he'll get rewarded with some great oral sex.

Standing on Mt. Olympus

In this position, he will feel like a Greek god, as he stands tall while you perform oral sex on your knees. Make activities on your knees the theme for the evening. Kissing, foreplay, oral sex, penetration positions, all acts of pleasure must be done on the knees. The most creative partner wins the title of God or Goddess for the night.

Two to Tango

Everyone can have fun at the same time. Here are a few positions for those who like to receive their pleasure from simultaneously having their genitals played with and their mouths full at the same time.

King and Queen of the Hill

Try a 69 position with either the male or female on top for a dominant flavor. Flip a coin and the winner gets the topside for 69 first, then switch.

69 Ways to Cuddle

Engulf your partner orally from a side-to-side position and experience the best of both oral worlds. Dare your lover to perform the best oral sex on you ever. They should pull out all the stops, using lubes, special tongue tricks, and sex toys. Whoever has their orgasm first must give their partner an erotic massage.

Olympic Weightlifting

Like an Olympic weightlifter, lift your partner up and hold them upside down as you both perform oral sex on each other. The point of this game is to do this once just to say that you did it!

Walk the Plank

Have one partner get in a reverse crab position, meaning they're on their hands and feet with their chest facing up, and the partner get on top of them for a modified 69 position. It's no secret you'll need to be in tiptop shape for this one. Use some flavored lube and see how long you can stay in this position.

Intercourse Position Games

What better way to keep the good times rolling than with penetration? Most couples like a little in and out action, and a variety of positions will keep things interesting and pleasurable. All of these position games can be utilized and enjoyed if you have the desire to test the waters outside your comfort zone.

Cowboy

This classic missionary position still gets the heart pumping with dominant and submissive alignments. Lying face to face, it features the cowboy on top and the partner beneath. The lover on top wears a cowboy hat and rides to their liking, from a slow trot to an all out gallop, and every speed in between.

Figure V

Try this spicy variation of missionary where one partner is on top and the bottom partner has their legs opened up wide in the shape of a V. The partner on the bottom has to try to touch the wall or headboard with their feet without help. Additional sexual treats are in order if successful.

Ride 'em Saucy Cowgirl

In this missionary position, she'll have the utmost control of the speed and depth of penetration as she is on top with edible oil or chocolate sauce on her nipples. The game is to see if her lover can catch them in his mouth while being ridden.

Reverse Saucy Cowgirl

Some like it hot while others like it flipped around. Here the cowgirl faces her partner's genitals for a different kind of ride.

Before she gets in the saddle, she can use a feather to tickle his testicles. If he laughs, he gets an extra ride.

Snoopy Style

Get in touch with the animal inside you and enjoy this Doggy-Style position from behind. While one partner is on all fours, the other enters them from behind. Have a bet on how many strokes it will take to orgasm. One way to cheat is to reach between your legs and fondle his scrotum to make him climax faster.

Puppy Pretzel is Doggy-Style with a twist. One person enters from behind while on their knees. The other wraps their legs around the back of their partner and pretzels them with their legs.

Downward Facing Good Doggy

Bring your yoga skills into this position as one partner is in downward dog position on all fours with straight arms and legs, and the other comes in from the rear. Bending forward can change up this position. Start with some naked yoga stretching and synchronized breathing and see how long you can concentrate on yoga before wanting to have sex.

Up Close and Personal

This position gets two people up close and personal as one partner enters from behind while laying on top pressing down on the other. The bottom partner can close their legs to tightly grip the penis as they are penetrated for a tight and snug fit during intercourse. For fun, attach a cock ring on the penis to give extra stimulation when gripping tightly. See if you can actually grip the ring with your legs.

The Sex Barrow

Start in a downward dog position and the person behind grabs their partner's thighs and lifts their legs off the floor while penetrating them. Try taking a few steps and make a bet on how many you can take. The winner gets an arm massage afterwards.

Froggy-Style

This position works well for partners with strong legs. While he is on his back, she squats down and sits on his penis. Then hop up and down or as much as your legs can take. While hopping, see how many times you can kiss your partner on the lips. This can heighten intimacy and add a fun time.

Toad-Style

Have one partner bent over on all fours while the other partner enters them from behind. How does this Toad-Style differ from Doggy-Style you may ask? The person behind is on their feet and typically the couple is having anal sex. Count how many times his scrotum hits the vulva and gently massage them for the same exact amount of times.

If you haven't noticed yet, all of the intercourse positions can be done vaginally or anally. You can choose which love hole you want to try.

Meditation Style

Use this Tantric inspired seated lap position to bring you and your partner closer together. Sit on top of his penis then wrap your legs around him and line up your faces and bodies for an intimate ride. Place a piece of fruit in your mouth to see if your partner can take it with their mouth. This will insure you are in perfect alignment.

The Wedding Walker

We're not walking down the aisle with this position, but it would make for an interesting ceremony! Pick up your partner with both arms while penetrating them as if you were going to carry them through the door after getting married.

Spoon Full of Sugar

This intimate position is for the lovers who enjoy facing one another while lying on their sides during penetration. Try to look at your partner throughout the entire lovemaking session. The first one to look away will provide an extra added something to the winner.

Backdoor Spooning

It doesn't mean you have to be utilizing the forbidden backdoor in this position, but you are spooning while having rear entry sex. But first, place a spoon in the freezer before you heat things up, and whoever comes first during your spooning position sex gets to tease their lover's hot spots with this icy utensil.

Scissor Twists

Try interlocking your legs like two pairs of scissors during penetration and test out your flexibility. You'll never look at a pair of scissors the same way again!

Kneeling Thrusts

This little variation goes a long way. One partner lies on their side while the other partner kneels and penetrates them hitting all the right spots.

Pillow Talk

Take the pillows from your bed and use them for other reasons besides resting your head. Pillows are a great way to alter the angle of entry or add comfort to any sexual position by placing them under your butt, back, head, tummy, thighs, or knees. See how many pillows you both can stack together to create a passion mount. The catch is to not use your hands.

With a couple of pillows under your butt, it helps to spread the legs easily so that your lover can have greater access to give you oral sex and deeper penetration.

Liberate Your Body

Sex cushions like the Liberator series are sturdy supportive pads that hold people in positions that might otherwise be difficult to maintain or perform. You can use one shape at a time, such as the Cube, Stage, Ramp, Wedge, or Scoop, or you can combine shapes like the Ramp and Wedge. Even better, the extra support leaves your hands free for something sexier like a courtesy reach around. These are available at Hustler retail stores or online. Use index cards to describe various positions, have your partner choose a card, and you create that position for added fun.

Queen For a Day

A Queening Stool is a crotchless seat for a partner to sit on while the oral sex genius performs from below. The stool holds weight and position so that getting and giving pleasure have all the focus. Combining pillows or Liberator cushions in the right way underneath the stool allows for penetration of the seated partner. Queening stools are available at www.fetishfurniturefactory.com.

If a Queening Stool peaks your interest, try the My Diletto self-pleasuring chair, a special chair with a custom built dildo attachment that penetrates the seated person as they rock forward. Find this chair at www.MyDiletto.com.

Sex Swings

Have a blast with a prop that makes you feel like Tarzan or Jane swinging on vines. Sex swings can be installed in any room to suspend a partner from the ceiling in a variety of gravity-defying positions. The swing supports the weight while you focus on more pleasurable activities. Some feel like a superhero in flight. Write fantasies about your favorite superhero, place them in a bag, and have your partner choose one to act out using the swing. You can find the Spinning Sex Swing, Trinity Sex Swing, Sportsheets Door Jam Sex Swing Sling, and the Adventure Industries Pleasure Swing online for purchase.

Rig Me Baby

Leg Riggings are tied around a person's ankles and go around the back of the shoulders to hold up the legs in the missionary position. Letting go of the need to hold up your legs might free you up to concentrate more on intimate things in the moment. Online adult sites also sell a variety of restraints from Sportsheets, Cal Exotics, Trinity Vibes, and Pipedreams.

Bulging Jeans

Take your favorite dildo and pair of jeans to make a sexy strap on. Just slide the dildo inside your jeans and only button the top button to create a hole for the dildo to come out of. Take a set of plastic rings and toss them at the dildo to see who can land the most. The winner gets to use the dildo anywhere they want.

Sexy Eyewear

Take a pair of swimming goggles and paint the insides with black paint. Allow it to dry and you have the perfect blindfold prop for the eyes. Play a sexy version of pin the tail on the donkey. Use your eyewear and no clothing. The winner picks their favorite position and keeps the eyewear on for more sensory fun.

Door Jam Cuffs

This clever prop is from Sportsheets. The tubing holds the door straps securely in place and won't damage doors, while the strong metal snaps secure the cuffs to the door straps so that you can have sex standing up while being restrained or restraining your lover. Add a feather tickler to challenge your lover's arousal. Give them a time limit of about 15 seconds, and if they last, give them an extra tug.

Hump

Hump is a game that teaches you and your lover about each other's libidos while traveling around the game board. Some cards offer lovemaking tips and others ask questions about your sexual likes and dislikes. The winner enjoys the reward of selecting three cards to interpret and act out during lovemaking. Hump is by Kheper Games and is available from Hustler stores and online.

8

Oral Sex Games— Licks and Kisses

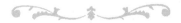

If you think oral sex is just a lick here and a suck there, get ready to turn up the creative volume with these oral sex games that will help you to reach levels of ecstasy you may not have known possible.

In this chapter, you are going to let your mouth explore your lover's loins and discover the immense pleasure that oral games can add to your relationship. Oral sex is one of the most intimate sexual acts you can do with your partner.

Oral Sex Games to Please a Woman

Cunnilingus is oral sex performed on a female, and it's one of the best ways for a woman to reach orgasm and experience ultimate sexual satisfaction. She'll love the playfulness of incorporating oral games into sex and you'll find that variety truly is the spice of life and love.

The Erotic Alphabet

Make a bet to see what letter your lady is going to reach her orgasm with. Then write the alphabet over her entire vulva with your tongue. Use the tip of your tongue from the top of her clitoris all the way down to the opening of her vagina. Make your tongue flat and wide when you cross the letter A. Then trace the letter B, which has a few more curves in it and will stimulate different parts of her vagina. Continue to slide and twist your tongue around her vulva as you spell the rest of the letters. Will she reach the big O before you do? The winner gets a cash prize.

Find Her U-Spot

By using your tongue as your guide, you have five minutes to find her U-spot—a small patch of sensitive erectile tissue located just above and on either side of the urethral opening (in other words it's her pee hole). The rules are for you to locate and lick it until she pushes you away. Your prize is a reciprocal five-minute licking on any hot spot you choose.

The Handyman

It's your duty to paint the fence using your tongue all the way from her anus to her clitoris with the flat of your tongue. She decides how many strokes she needs to be satisfied and that the job is done well. If you finish the job the way she likes it, you win a romantic dinner followed by erotic pampering. If you fail to finish the job, you must wash the windows using your tongue as a windshield wiper from side to side on her vulva until she tells you to stop.

What Time Is It?

Play a game that challenges the time it takes for your lover to climax from oral sex. Estimate the time it takes her in minutes. If you are less than one minute off, then you win a sexual pleasure of your choice.

The Clitoral Truth

Play truth or dare with your partner and use female oral sex as your prize. Ask your partner sexual trivia such as, what's my favorite position? For a dare, dare your lover to perform your favorite oral sex technique on you for at least two minutes, then continue the game.

How imaginative can you be when it comes to safer sex with female oral play? There are female condoms and dental dams of course, but you can make your own creative barrier by cutting male condoms open or making a latex glove into a mouth dam. All you need to do is cut off the four fingers, leave the thumb (for your tongue later), and cut down the side opposite from the thumb. Presto! You made a dental dam with tongue action.

Chinese Field Goal

You'll need plastic chopsticks, a steady hand, and a talented tongue for this game. Place each chopstick along the outer edge of your woman's vaginal lips, then use your thumb and finger to gently roll each fold of skin around the chopstick so that it resembles goal posts. Your tongue becomes the football and you must score at least three field goals by placing it between the posts in five minutes. If you win, you are a hero, but if you lose then no oral sex for you for a week.

Water Her Flower

Stand her up and imagine that her legs are the stems and her vagina is a beautiful delicate flower such as a tulip, lily, rosebud, or pussy willow that you are going to moisten with your tongue. She has to guess what kind of flower you are watering by your actions. If she guesses correctly, buy her a bunch of the same flowers.

Oral Sex Games to Please a Man

If you've ever heard of the word fellatio, then you know it means oral sex performed on a penis, also known as a blow job. As much fun as a blow job can be, sometimes adding the right amount of gamesmanship can turn a good one into a great one just by adding an exciting game with an arousing twist.

Condom Fashion Show

Purchase as many different kinds of condoms as you can that include a variety of shapes, colors, scents, flavors, styles, and materials. Then see how many you can put on him before he loses his erection.

A good trick to putting a condom on a man and keeping him hard is to put it on with your mouth. Turn it so that the receptacle end is inside your mouth, and the rolled rim is in front of your teeth, but behind your lips and then slide it on, pushing the condom onto the head of his penis with your lips. Finally, roll the condom down the shaft of the penis with your lips.

Lipstick Magic

Take three different colors of lipstick and assign an oral sex style to each color. For example, when you wear pink it means oral sex with no hands, red is for oral with one hand on his testes, and plum is for oral with one finger in the anus.

A Man's Favorite Alarm Clock

Make a bet that you can get your man hard and perform fellatio on him before he wakes up. You have one week to achieve this. Grab your cell phone and take a snapshot as evidence that you got him hard while he slept. What does the winner get? Dinner at your favorite restaurant and afterwards, the choice to give or receive oral sex any way you want.

The Fly and the Frog

Put his penis between your breasts and make a bet to see how many inches of his penis you can suck at the same time. If you win, he has to be your servant for one night.

Flagpole Toss

Play a ring toss game on a man's erect penis with female panties. You get 10 panty tosses from five feet away while he is standing and erect. For each toss landed, your prize is a good licking in any position that you desire, until you say that you've had enough.

Deep Throat

How deep can you go? Bet your partner how many mouth strokes you can deep throat his penis. If you reach the number of strokes you bet on, you win and can choose the way he ejaculates. If he wins, then he chooses the way he gets to shoot.

Think deep throating isn't for you? Try a sore throat lozenge to numb the back of your throat before going down on him. It takes the tickle away and gives you a little something extra in the deep throat department. Wait at least 15 minutes after you've finished the lozenge; otherwise his penis may feel the numbness, too.

Double Trouble

Think you have what it takes to engulf your man's pride and joy? Challenge your partner to a duel and see if you can place his penis and testicles in your mouth at the same time. If you can, you win a prize that you wished for and wrote down on a piece of paper before starting the game. If you lose, then keep practicing.

Oral Sex Games for Fun Couples

Couples who play together, stay together. These games will add more sizzle and are for all sexual orientations whether you are dating, living together, just married, or in a long-term relationship.

Your Highness

Treat your lover like a King or a Queen when they have done something that deserves a reward. Tell them to sit upon a throne to be orally pampered. Actually, they can sit anywhere like the edge of the bed, a chair, sofa, or even on the stairs as you kneel before him or her and service them orally.

Try this icebreaker for a fun addition to any game. Put ice in your mouth before or during oral sex to give your partner a cool sensation. Or try sipping on hot tea beforehand to get them hot and bothered in a good way.

Sexy Spelling Bee

Challenge your partner to a sexual spelling bee and have the oral sex giver spell sexual words on the receiver's genitals. Slowly spell the naughty words with a pointy tongue and reward your lover with at least five minutes of oral pleasure when they guess the word.

Picasso's Paintbrush

Face each other naked with legs wide apart and have a contest to draw each other's genitals in a 15-minute time limit. You can use paint, crayons, colored pencils, or markers. The winner is the most artistic expression of their lover's vagina or penis and the prize is a steamy night of passion.

Knocking on the Backdoor

Have a silent staring contest with your lover that includes making faces and anything to get your partner to laugh. The loser is the person who laughs first, and they must give an oral tongue bath that ends up knocking on the backdoor. Give erotic shivers by licking down the spine swirling your tongue as you trail your way toward the buttocks.

Balloon Blower

Play a game of water balloon toss with your lover. After each toss and catch, take a small step backward and continue until the balloon bursts. The loser must give oral sex to the winner until they climax.

The Lube Job

Oral sex can be even tastier with the addition of flavored lubes, such as strawberry, cherry, tangerine, pineapple, and chocolate. Put a dab of lube on different parts of your body and see how many flavors your lover can guess correctly by licking them all off.

Head or Tails

To avoid arguments about who gets to receive oral pleasure first, flip a coin. Challenge your partner to a tournament of three flips and see who gets lucky by getting heads more than tails.

For a sneaky guarantee, use a magician's double-sided heads coin. If you get caught, you're in big trouble, so refer to Chapter 10 for ideas on your "punishment."

Oral Dancing

Have a dance contest. For her, spread her inner labia lips and dart your pointy tongue in and out of her vaginal opening rhythmically as if you were dancing the Cha Cha. So the movements would be: Slow, slow, quick, quick, slow, slow, slow, quick, quick, slow and keep on doing this until she tells you to stop. Then turn the tables and oral dance the Cha Cha on his penis.

Musical Genius

Suck on your lover's perineum as if you are playing a harmonica, and be sure to add some humming sounds for extra stimulation and vibration. Can he or she guess the song you're playing? Name that tune never had such an oral edge. The receiver who guesses the right tune gets to choose what they want to do on their next date night.

Oral Gambler

Roll a pair of dice to see if you are the giver or receiver of oral pleasure. The amount added up from your roll determines how many minutes of facial intercourse you get. Roll a 2 and a 6, that's 8 minutes. Roll pairs and you get double the number. Roll a snake eyes (two 1's) and you get triple the number on your next roll. Roll a 7 or 11 and you lose, no face pumping tonight.

Aces for Analingus

Take a walk on the open-minded side as you take a deck of cards and deal all the shuffled cards face down. Turn over your cards and whoever has more aces gets their anus licked. (To practice safer sex, be sure to use a barrier such as plastic food wrap or a dental dam.)

Simultaneous Oral Games

Reaching the "big O" at the same time can be a body-melting experience and these games will help you increase your arousal levels so that you can climax at the same time.

The Tortoise and the Hare

Instead of racing to see who finishes first, why not finish together? Get in your favorite 69 position and work together to cum together. If you normally pop quickly, tell your lover to stop and give you a break. If you normally need more time, make sure you get that extra attention.

Crazy 69's

Just like you would play the card game, Crazy Eights, change it up to Crazy Sixes and Nines. Play one round with the number six and then play the next round with the number nine. If the score is 1 to 1, play a tie breaking round for the winning prize. The winner gets to choose whether they are on top or bottom for a hot and steamy 69 session.

The Oral Buzz

Get into a 69 sideways position and use a small vibrator to stimulate your lover's clitoris, testes, or anus while you are licking them at the same time. The game is to move into the man or woman on top 69 position just before you both orgasm simultaneously.

The Screaming O LING-O vibrating tongue rings go on the base of your tongue for enhanced oral play. They are available at Hustler stores and online.

Computer Love

Do you Skype or webcam? Have your partner sneak in a quick oral sex session on you as you have a televised chat with someone. The game is coming as close to getting caught without getting caught. Make sure you position the camera high enough so your cam buddy doesn't see anything, like the top of your partner's head sneaking into the picture. Unless that's what you want!

{ Have fun! }

9

Sex Fantasies and Role-Playing Games

In this chapter, you'll discover the exciting world of sex games with fantasy and role play. Sharing and living out these fantasies will expand your sexual boundaries, improve your intimate communication, and create new memories.

Role-playing sexual fantasies are healthy, fun, and natural. It works for couples dating or for those in a committed relationship of any orientation. Fantasies can rekindle passion, raise a diminished libido, boost intimacy, act as an exciting avenue of escape, heighten enjoyment of sex, open you up to new activities, and can turn sex into adult play.

Sharing Fantasy Games

The goal of sharing fantasies is for the two of you to experience as many role-playing characters as you can. When couples act out each other's fantasies, they gain a better understanding of what the other wants, needs, and desires. So take a chance and let your lover in on your naughty secret thoughts and take turns initiating these fantasy games. There are no losers in these games, only winners.

Eight Fantasy Dates

Not since Chanukah has there been eight days of pleasure like this. Have you and your partner write a list of eight sex fantasies you have and rank them in order based on which is most exciting. After you have your lists, agree to spend the next eight days sharing them with each other. Each day, write one page on each of your fantasies and share it with your partner. On the ninth day, place the pages in a bag and take turns randomly selecting one at a time to live out. With eight days of build up, the ninth day and on is sure to please.

Fantasy Fortune Telling

Try this verbal fantasy game to test both your creativity and imagination. Start off with a timer and give each person 20 seconds. Flip a coin and the winner will begin to describe a sex fantasy scenario, such as a Threesome or Anal fantasy. After 20 seconds, switch and the other partner will continue the fantasy for another 20 seconds. Do this for five turns and see what erotic ideas you come up with. At the end, you can decide if it's a fantasy you want to live out.

Building Blocks of Pleasure

Start by having one partner write one paragraph to begin a fantasy and e-mail it to the other partner who must add one more fantasy paragraph by the end of the day and e-mail it back. (Be sure to only use your personal e-mail accounts!) Continue adding paragraphs each day until the end of the week, when you should have 14 paragraphs combined. When you've completed your story, you can read it aloud in your sexiest voices.

If your partner starts a fantasy about something like bondage and that's not a turn-on for you, change it to another fantasy such as having a private erotic dancer who was able to unbind him or herself.

Fantasy Fun Cards

Write down all your sexual fantasies on a stack of cards and get your lover to do the same. Then each of you sort all of your cards into two separate piles: one is fantasies to turn into reality, perhaps having sex in a public place, or being a sex slave, and the other is fantasies to remain only as fantasies, maybe it's having group sex or having sex with someone of the same sex. Expressing your sexual fantasies can be a huge part of foreplay, or it can be the main event.

Paint a Picture

Play a sexy version of the game Pictionary where you and your partner take turns drawing different fantasies. Each person will get five turns to try and guess what the other is drawing in under a minute. You can draw stick figures or sketch drawings of your fantasies, such as a Playboy Bunny Rock Star, Sexy Maid, or Butler.

Fantasy Charades

Play a game of fantasy charades where you get to act out your favorite sexual fantasies without speaking. See if your partner can guess what you are trying to tell them through your actions and movements.

Use as many props in Fantasy Charades as you can find to help your partner guess your fantasy. For example, if you have a cop fantasy, get some handcuffs. If your fantasy is being a doctor or nurse, get some latex gloves, and if your fantasy is being Little Red Riding Hood, get a red cape with a picnic basket.

The Funny Pages

Draw 10 boxes and create a comic strip about your fantasy. Be as descriptive as you like and share your comic with your partner. Make sure your pictures have a beginning, middle, and an end. For example, you can draw a character that is a Masked Lover and write: "I can rescue you from the menace of the city." Then draw a picture of the damsel in distress crying for help, and so on.

Chased by the Paparazzi

Pretend you and your lover are a popular celebrity couple going to a red carpet event. Rent a limo for the night and put on your sexiest dress or suit for a hot night on the town. Stock the limo with bubbly and sexy music and go out to dinner, clubs, and just drive around feeling like the paparazzi is watching your every move. Call each other by your celebrity names and steam up those backseat windows with some hot sex before the night is through.

Fantasy Sexting

Text your lover a sexual fantasy that you are too shy to talk about face to face, like a Naughty Schoolgirl fantasy. You can text, "I want you to put on your short school girl skirt, tight button down blouse, and knee highs." Your partner's response may be: "Ok, are you going to bend me over your knee for a spanking?" Response from the fantasizer: "First you're going to suck my lollipop, then I'm going to pull your panties down and spank you." Keep the fantasy sexting going until you are in the same room and you'll be so hot for each other that your fantasy reality will sizzle.

Hot Male Fantasy Games

Men's fantasies are often more sexually explicit and visually arousing with specific themes. Here are some fantasy games to satisfy his thirst for something sexy.

Ménage à Trois

Having sex with two women at the same time is one of the biggest fantasies for guys, but both of you must agree to want to act it out. And there is an alternative; you can make this fantasy exciting for him by creating a threesome scenario while you're having sex together. Describe what the other woman looks like (make her the opposite of you) and ask him to describe what he wants her to do to you both. Use plenty of dirty talk and he may not even realize the difference between fantasy and reality.

The Seducer

Men enjoy being the sexual conquerors and it's sure to come out in their sexual fantasies. From Casanova to Don Juan, men have been inspired to be playful and seductive creatures. Agree to act out a seduction scenario at a local bar, and be sure to arrive separately. When he arrives, he should act out his most suave moves to seduce you in public. It can be a seduction line, sending over a drink from the other side of the bar or an obvious wink from a distance and motion to come to him. Let the actor inside fuel this fantasy.

Dom Da Dom Dom

Many men love to express their dominant sides with their fantasies. Have some necessary accessories on hand such as sexy black leather, latex or satin clothes, gloves, scarf, blindfold, and whip or paddle. Have him tell you that you need to be punished for bad behavior and let him take you somewhere where he can be completely in charge. His body language should be authoritative, shoulders back, head up, and hands on hips with a confident attitude as he tells you exactly how to satisfy him. If you don't comply, you'll get a good spanking.

Yellow Submarine

Some men enjoy living out their submissive fantasies as well. Be the dominant and let him be at your submissive call. How do you like to be served by your submissive? Whether it's cooking for you, pleasuring you, or bathing you with his tongue, a good slave always gets rewarded.

The Knight in Shining Armor

Many men have a Knight in Shining Armor fantasy and here's a fun game for him to act it out. Drive to a crowded area and pull over to the side to make it appear that your car has broken down. That's when he comes to the rescue as he drives up just a few moments later and looks under the hood. Miraculously, he fixes the car and you give him a huge passionate kiss, then proceed to reward him with sexual bliss back at his place, or in the backseat.

Mr. Grandiose

Men love to hear they are the greatest lover their partner has ever had. And who wouldn't like the ego boost? Live out a sexual fantasy where he can do no wrong in the bedroom. Give him constant praise in graphic detail, scream and pant like a porn star, and make it clear that he is the best lover you've ever had.

Sexy Female Fantasy Games

Fantasies for women can range from highly romantic and seductive to dirty and dangerous. These fantasy games for her are sure to add a new dimension in the bedroom.

Seduce Me

Many females have their own seduction fantasy of having their partner whisk them away to an erotic, orgasmic place. Create a fantasy where she is being seduced by you. She says no, but your persistence and smooth talking turns her on until she can't help herself but to give in to your sexual desires and advances.

Set the mood for seduction and stimulate all her senses by playing sensual music, having candlelight, comfy pillows, her favorite drink, and tasty treats.

Masochist Mayhem

Of all the kinks out there, you'll find that some women enjoy having some pain with pleasure. Start by coming up with three different light masochistic sexual acts she may enjoy, such as having her clothes or underwear torn off, being spanked, having her hair pulled or being restrained with your hands during sex. Give them each a try and see what she likes.

The Pampered Princess

Many women enjoy feeling like a princess for a day. So create a fantasy scenario where she has every sexual wish granted while being pampered. If that means sending her to a spa, then taking her shopping, followed by a romantic meal before making passionate love to her, then you must grant her royal wishes and treat her like the princess that she is.

Romantic Rendezvous

Women often have dreams of being romanced and fantasies of intimate moments with their partner. Make the dream a reality by giving her the romantic night she's always imagined. Shower the bed with rose petals, sip champagne while taking a bubble bath, feed her chocolate-dipped strawberries, and become the person that authors write erotic novels about. Be the romantic lover that she always fantasized about and create a memory she won't soon forget.

Three's Not a Crowd

It's not unusual for women to fantasize about having sex with other women now and again. But in this fantasy sex game, her lover can only play voyeur until she gives him permission to join in. With these rules the woman is in control of the fantasy game without feeling jealous and he gets his Ménage à Trois fantasy fulfilled.

Some women fantasize about having a threesome with two men, and that's something to explore with her by discussing the pros and cons first.

Dominatrix

Some women fantasize about being more dominant in the bedroom. They enjoy taking control and want to dominate their lover as a way to unleash their innermost desires. Have her list her three most powerful dominant desires like talking dirty, being on top, digging her fingernails into your back during sex, or just tying you up. Then let her do all three.

Couples Role-Playing Games

Because so many men and women have top, bottom, dominant, and submissive fantasies, included here are these fantasies for everyone to enjoy.

Comic Play

Live out your comic dreams with this fantasy game. Purchase a comic book with your favorite character, and dress up and act out the scenes with your partner. However, you also must include a sex scene that's not in the comic. Place it at an opportune time, as a reward for a good deed.

Some comic book characters you can role play include Superman, The Hulk, Wonder Woman, Punisher, Cat Woman, and Poison Ivy.

Call Me Anytime

Play a naughty game of phone sex operator with your partner. Have him or her call you for some sexual TLC and release. Describe what you're wearing and how you are touching yourself, as you get more and more aroused. Make sure you use your phone sex voice and add all the right sounds to get your partner off, as any good operator would.

Strangers in the Night

It's the danger that puts the naughty in this fantasy. Go out in disguise wearing a wig, hat, fake moustache, or dress out of character and go to a public place to pretend you've never met before. Flirt and seduce each other, then go to a hotel for a one-night stand. Don't exchange names or numbers as you make this anonymous, stranger fantasy come true.

Freeze or I'll Shoot

Dress up as a police officer and come home to find your partner robbing the house. This burglar needs to be arrested and punished. Instead of sending him or her to jail, you decide to give them house arrest and teach them a lesson in the bedroom.

Paging Doctor Love

Have one partner be the doctor and the other is the patient who lays on the examination table and shows parts of his or her body that need more attention. The good doctor does whatever is needed to make sure their patient leaves cured.

Pay for Play

Set up a scene where one partner is a sex worker and the other is paying for their sexual services. Act out the entire transaction, from the phone call asking about the various services they offer all the way through to the final payment.

Some sex services you can offer your lover can include a hand job, blow job, vibrator show, Love at the Y (cunnilingus), half and half (half oral and half intercourse), and around the world (oral, intercourse, and anal sex).

Dancing for Tips

Take turns making some extra money by showing your hot moves to your lover. As your partner nears nudity, shower him or her with more money by stuffing it in their underwear. This is one strip club that your partner will surely like.

Movie Star Madness

Get into character and reenact your favorite sex scenes from movies. A few good movies to check out for this are: *Shortbus, The Pornographer, Intimacy, Brokeback Mountain, 9-1/2 Weeks,* and *In the Realm of the Senses.*

Under the Midnight Moon

Take a walk on the wild side and role play exhibitionism and public sex. Sneak away with your partner to a secluded place where you won't get caught and ravage your lover under the midnight moon. The rush of being outdoors just might be an intoxicating adventure you'll never forget.

Lights, Camera, Action!

Grab your movie camera and act out a porn scene by filming you and your lover as porn stars. Set up your tripod or connect your camera to the TV so you can watch your moves.

For a fantasy twist, be the director and direct your lover in a masturbation scene.

Taboo Fantasy Games

Some fantasy and role-playing games are way over the top and realistically impractical, but in fantasyland anything is possible through the power of suggestion. These fantasies don't need to be fulfilled, but they can make for some freaky sex games when you pretend you are doing them during sex with your lover.

- Sex while riding a roller coaster
- Sex with your best friend's spouse
- Having sex as a virgin
- Sex as the opposite gender
- Sex with a celebrity
- Sex with a relative
- Sex on skis
- Sex in space
- Orgy sex

With all fantasies, the only limits are the ones that you and your lover put on them. If you want your sex life to be more playful, then take a risk and share all your craziest fantasies with your lover, and it might just be the missing ingredient for the best sex you've ever had.

Have fun!

10

Power Play Games

In the sex community, BDSM are four letters that stand for six words—Bondage, Discipline, Domination, Submission, Sadism, and Masochism. It's a playground teeming with games to utilize the exchange of power to heighten pleasure and tantalize the senses.

In this chapter, we will explore the titillating world of these power exchange sex games where you and your partner trade off being sexually dominant and submissive to one another. You will need an open mind, mutually trusting hearts, and a bit of imagination to let these games be fun and exciting for you and your partner. Some other key ingredients include trust, respect, consent, good negotiation skills, honesty, and great communication. Some of the sex games may include being tied up or blindfolded, so having a solid sense of trusting your partner to have your best interests in hand is important.

Bondage

Bondage is restraining or restricting a person's ability to move. You may not realize that you already enjoy bondage in lighter forms. Have you ever held down your partner or been held down? Maybe you took a silk scarf or his work tie and used them to blindfold or restrain your partner? Do you have a pair of handcuffs in your bag of sexy tricks? Each of these are versions of bondage and power exchange in mild forms.

It's important to pick some safe words that you and your partner agree will immediately stop the power play and let you check in with each other. Common words used correspond to a traffic light, red for stop, yellow for stay where you are, and green for keep going!

Prisoner of Love

Make a bet to see who knows exactly what time it is without looking at a watch or clock. The person closest to the right time can choose to be the prisoner or the captor of love. The captor restrains the prisoner's hands and feet with scarves, stockings, neckties, rope, or cuffs, so that they are powerless. Then make passionate love to your partner until one or both of you reach orgasm.

Blind Love

Flip a coin to see who is going to be blindfolded and then lead your lover to the bed. Undress and ravish him or her with total abandon, which should be easy because they can't see you.

Cops and Robbers

Cops always put handcuffs on those naughty robbers. Buy a pair of fuzzy, padded handcuffs, or whatever type you prefer, to use to "arrest" your lover for taking the last cookie, beer, the remote, or whatever you deem as a theft. Take turns being the cop and the robber.

Teepee Your Partner

Wrap your partner's wrists and ankles in toilet paper for a lighter, fluffier restraint. While he or she is restrained, undress yourself and tease your lover to the point they can't stay restrained any longer and have to rip free of the restraints. Take turns being the one restrained.

Playful Plastic Wrap

Time to venture into the kitchen to give plastic wrap more to do than covering leftovers. Take turns wrapping different parts of your partner's body with this clear plastic restraint. Just remember that any restraint can be too tight, so check in with your partner for feedback.

Cowboy and Cowgirl Rope Ties

Rope can be used for restraints. It's always a good idea to learn easy rope ties that make for easy and quick adjusting. Those with a sailor's background or scout badges in knot tying from their childhood will have a leg up on the rope bondage play.

When choosing a rope for restraints, use solid braid rope made from nylon, hemp, or cotton clothesline and measure your arm span for the size.

Mouth Bondage

Pick a number between 1 and 10 and write it down. The person who picked the number closest to the written down number takes a pair of underwear and places it inside their partner's mouth to make a gag. This will keep them from talking back or giving you any lip while you explore sexual pleasure with them. Breathing through the nose is essential and the ability to remove the gag at anytime is crucial.

Pantyhose Straitjacket

A naughty slave should be ordered to fold his or her arms while you wrap several pairs of pantyhose around their body, while they are lying down on a bed. Don't cover their nose or mouth as you are going to straddle their face so they can lick you while they breathe through their nose. Be sure to remove the straitjacket after they've given you a good licking.

Discipline, Dominance, and Submission

Do you like to be in charge in the bedroom, the dominant, or does it turn you on to be punished, the submissive? A dominant can train a submissive with discipline to behave in a certain way, in the name of sexual fun. More fun happens when the rules aren't met, and the best punishments come from your imagination and can be inspired from some of these power exchange games.

Scavenger Hunt

Collect some basic items from around the house and put them out for your partner to find when he or she gets home. The items will be used sexually, for example ordinary dental floss can make for great nipple or testicle bondage. An electric toothbrush can be used to stimulate the inside of the thighs or tickle like crazy in between the toes.

Punishment Box

Keep a secret box of "punishments" to use on your lover when it's time for some fun. Have a set of cards with erotic punishments written on each one so that you can pick one randomly. Punishments can range from being tied up, blindfolded, and deprived of orgasm, spanked, or humiliated by walking around naked wearing a leash.

The Sensual Slave

Using a dartboard, give each other 10 chances to hit a bullseye. The loser becomes an erotic slave for an entire six-hour evening. Each bullseye reduces the time by 30 minutes. Even if you have an expert dart thrower who hits 10 bullseyes, you're still guaranteed one hour of slave time.

An erotic slave can do anything you ask of them from licking your feet, masturbating in front of you, to bringing you a beer.

The XXX Ending

When your partner has been a bad boy or girl, restrain their hands and ankles, then punish them by pleasuring them almost to orgasm. When they're ready to erupt, pull back and keep stimulating them and withdrawing before orgasm three times until they beg for the mighty O. Have mercy on your submissive by eventually giving them their orgasm.

The Punisher

Put a small object in one of your hands behind your back and ask your partner to guess which hand it's in. If they are right, then they are the punisher who gets to punish you with any one of these disciplines: nipple pinching, spanking, hair pulling, humiliation, or the silent treatment.

Ping Pong Paddling

All you need is a ping pong table and a competitive edge. Play ping pong in the nude and keep score. Serve an ace, you get to choose to spank or be spanked once with a paddle. Win the game, you get a spanking session of your choice. Win the best of three games and you get to incorporate a restraint of your choice with the ping pong paddle.

Brushing Your Backside

Grab your favorite hair brush and a coin to flip. Heads you spank your lover with the brush, tails you get spanked. Use the flat side of your brush to get spanked when you lose one time. Use the bristle side to get spanked if you lose twice in a row.

The Ravager

Call or text your partner and instruct them to put on some old clothes that can be torn or cut off, because when you get home, you're going to throw him or her on the bed and ravage them forcefully.

Public Discipline

Take turns sending each other out in public or to work wearing a piece of your underwear as a reminder of who is in control.

Sadism and Masochism

A sadist enjoys inflicting painful sensations onto their partner while receiving pain turns on a masochist. You can make the sensations as mild or intense as your hearts desire. These types of games are the perfect playground for pain and pleasure enthusiasts.

Corporate Flogging

Play a game of strip blackjack with your partner. Whoever loses their clothes first gets the honor of being flogged on their bare buttocks with a pillowcase folded lengthwise. Keep count of the number of 21's and blackjacks each person gets and have those be special "double" floggings on both cheeks.

Locker Room Jock Play

Choose a sporting event and place a bet on who wins. The winner of the bet gets to lightly whip their partner. Create a homemade whip with a small hand towel and erotically whip your partner. Start off gently and learn the difference between snapping your wrist rapidly versus slow follow through.

Avoid hitting the face, ears, spine, hips, kidneys, and the tailbone located at the end of the spine where it curves into the anus. These are no spanking zones.

What's Your Number?

Next time you have sex in the Doggy-Style position, ask your partner if they want to be punished for being naughty. If they say "Yes," ask how many spanks they think that they can take? If they tell you to stop before the number, they lose and must please you in any manner that you desire.

Chinese Caning

Use chopsticks to "drum" a tune on your partner's butt and have him or her guess what you're playing. Give a hint by humming the tune along with your drum playing.

Have fun with your Chinese take-out. Take two chopsticks and tie two rubber bands around each edge
to join the chopsticks. Insert a nipple in between the
chopsticks. Now you have yourself homemade nipple
clamps. The tighter or looser you tie the rubberbands,
the more or less pressure the clamp has.

Painter's Touch

Buy watercolor paint and use your artistic skills for a sexy purpose. Have you and your partner compete in a painting for pleasure contest. Pick a sexy S/M scene, like tit torture, whipping, ice
play, testicle clamping, and paint it. The person who paints the
best picture gets to enact their scene and chooses the roles.

Manicure Heaven

Have a paper airplane making contest and see which plane
can stay flying the longest. The winner gets to trade in their
wings for nails. Your partner can be tied up or not as you use
your nails to scratch their back, arms, thighs, and everywhere
in between. Start off light and work your way up to heavier
scratches if your partner gives you the okay. Try scratching in
unique patterns to change up the sensation (up/down, circular,
wavy patterns, zigzag, etc.).

Playful Pinching

Ask your partner to answer an intimate question that they may
or may not know about you. If they answer correctly, they can
choose to pinch or be pinched on their buttocks for one minute. If
they answer incorrectly, you get to pinch away on their backside.

Take pinching to the next level. Use household clothespins to pinch your partner's nipples, testicles, labia, or any other part of their body that they want to have pinched.

Vampire's Bite

How long can your partner withstand a vampire bite? Make a bet as to how many seconds and see if you can withstand your partner's vampire bite anywhere that you choose on your body. If you last as long as you bet, the prize is oral sex, without the biting.

Wrestle Mania

Challenge your partner to a nude wrestling match and experience foreplay the Greco-Roman way. For an added twist, consider greasing yourself up with oil and incorporating aspects of bondage. Would wrestling blindfolded change the dynamic? Try and find out.

Bags of Kink

Take two bags and fill each of them with two different power play items. One bag is for Bondage restraints such as handcuffs, toilet paper, belts, neckties, rope, and scarves. The other bag is for Discipline and Punishment items such as a ruler, a paddle, nipple clamps, or clothes pegs. Pick one item from each bag to have your own power play trifecta. The more additions you add to each bag, the better and the winner is he or she who can use everything from both bags.

Take a cue from the gay community and explore hanky codes. A black one means heavy S/M, blue means oral sex, pink means tit torture. Placing the hanky in the back left pocket means you are the active/giver and the right pocket means you are the passive/receiver. What colors best represent your deepest, darkest desires?

Lusty Shopping Spree

Go with your partner to a dollar store and each fill up your own baskets with 10 items to use for power exchange games. For example, a spatula for caning, pantyhose for blindfolding, clothespins for pinching, bobbypins for scratching, an oven mitt for spanking, and tape for tying. After 15 minutes of shopping, get together and compare. The person to reach 10 items first wins.

Top and Bottom Satisfaction

Take turns switching between being a Top and a Bottom so that you can be a dominant one day and a submissive the next. As a Top, you can take away your slave's senses to make any punishment experience more intense. Take away their sense of sight with a blindfold, remove their sense of touch by restraining them, and deprive them of hearing with earplugs or earmuffs. Now you can stroke your lover's body with ice or any other textures.

The Sexy Little Book of

KAMA SUTRA

Take your love to erotic new depths

Ron Louis and Dave Copeland

Touches lightly on the philosophy of the Kama Sutra and focuses on the pure principles and techniques of ultimate gratification.

ISBN: 978-1-61564-133-8

The Sexy Little Book of

ORAL PLEASURE

Send your lover over the moon

Ava Cadell, Ph.D., Ed.D.

Packed with tips, tricks, and techniques for giving—and receiving—over-the-top pleasure in the "oral tradition."

ISBN: 978-1-61564-134-5

Have fun!

penguin.com